A Guide to
CHILD HEA

Warning

If you are in doubt, worried or uncertain about the diagnosis you should seek medical advice. This book is not intended to be used as an alternative to the advice of physicians. You should consult a physician about any symptoms which may require diagnosis or treatment.

A guide to
CHILD HEALTH

A practical guide to all
common problems
from birth to adolescence

Dr Vernon Coleman

Routledge & Kegan Paul

London, Melbourne and Henley

To my mother and father

First published in 1984 by
Routledge & Kegan Paul plc
39 Store Street, London WC1E 7DD, England,
464 St Kilda Road, Melbourne,
Victoria 3004, Australia and
Broadway House, Newtown Road,
Henley-on-Thames, Oxon RG9 1EN, England
Set in Rockwell by Columns of Reading
and printed in Great Britain by
T.J. Press (Padstow) Ltd, Padstow, Cornwall

British Library Cataloguing in Publication Data

Coleman, Vernon

A guide to child health.
1. Children—Care and hygiene
I. Title
613'.0432'0240431 RJ61

ISBN 0-7100-9632-1
ISBN 0-7102-0269-5 (pbk)

Contents

Note

Except where it would be obviously inappropriate I have used only the male pronoun in this book. I have done this simply to avoid confusion and unnecessary repetition.

Major warning signs

You must ask for professional advice if your child:

– cannot be roused.

– has any severe pain.

– has any pain which is unexplained and which persists.

– has any pain which is unexplained and which recurs.

– is losing weight.

– is bleeding from anything other than a minor cut, nose bleed, etc.

– needs to take home medicines regularly or for five days or more.

– has a poor appetite for five days or more.

– has a lump or swelling you can't explain.

– has been hit on the head.

– has been unconscious.

– has a lump, wart or skin blemish which has changed size or colour or bled.

– has a paralysis of any kind.

– wants to stay in bed.

– has developed new symptoms since starting medical treatment.

– has mental symptoms such as confusion or hallucinations.

– cries a lot.

Emergency notes

1 When asking emergency services to visit at night give landmarks and leave all lights switched on.

2 It is often quicker to use your own transport. Drive carefully and do not pass red lights. If possible take a healthy passenger with you to help with the patient.

3 Keep your doctor's address and telephone number and the address of your nearest hospital on this page.

Dealing with emergencies

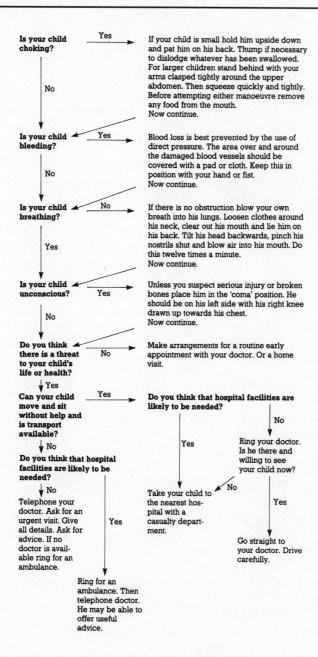

Is your child choking? — Yes →

If your child is small hold him upside down and pat him on his back. Thump if necessary to dislodge whatever has been swallowed. For larger children stand behind with your arms clasped tightly around the upper abdomen. Then squeeze quickly and tightly. Before attempting either manoeuvre remove any food from the mouth.
Now continue.

No ↓

Is your child bleeding? ← Yes →

Blood loss is best prevented by the use of direct pressure. The area over and around the damaged blood vessels should be covered with a pad or cloth. Keep this in position with your hand or fist.
Now continue.

No ↓

Is your child breathing? ← No →

If there is no obstruction blow your own breath into his lungs. Loosen clothes around his neck, clear out his mouth and lie him on his back. Tilt his head backwards, pinch his nostrils shut and blow air into his mouth. Do this twelve times a minute.
Now continue.

Yes ↓

Is your child unconscious? ← Yes →

Unless you suspect serious injury or broken bones place him in the 'coma' position. He should be on his left side with his right knee drawn up towards his chest.
Now continue.

No ↓

Do you think there is a threat to your child's life or health? ← No →

Make arrangements for a routine early appointment with your doctor. Or a home visit.

↓ Yes

Can your child move and sit without help and is transport available? — Yes →

Do you think that hospital facilities are likely to be needed?

↓ No

Do you think that hospital facilities are likely to be needed?

No →

Yes ↓

Ring your doctor. Is he there and willing to see your child now?

↓ No

Telephone your doctor. Ask for an urgent visit. Give all details. Ask for advice. If no doctor is available ring for an ambulance.

Yes →

Take your child to the nearest hospital with a casualty department. — No

Yes ↓

Go straight to your doctor. Drive carefully.

↓ Yes

Ring for an ambulance. Then telephone doctor. He may be able to offer useful advice.

A-Z of common problems

To use this part of the book effectively simply look up the symptom that is worrying you. In the appropriate section you'll find details of what you can and cannot do safely at home, which bits and pieces of traditional advice to follow and which to ignore. You'll also find advice on just when to ask for professional advice – and how to make sure that you understand what is being done. These sections are all designed: to help you before you need medical advice, to help you decide when you need medical advice, and to help you when you have sought professional help.

Abdominal pain

What causes it?
Most parents think of appendicitis when their children complain of abdominal pain. Most doctors think of appendicitis too. When I was a medical student I remember being told by a very experienced physician that if a child complains of abdominal pain then a diagnosis of appendicitis should always be assumed. I even remember being told that a doctor who diagnoses appendicitis every time he sees a child with abdominal pain will probably have a better diagnostic record than the doctor who tried to produce a specific, individual diagnosis on each occasion!

The truth, however, is that although appendicitis is certainly the *commonest* single serious disease causing abdominal pain it certainly isn't the *only* disease. There are dozens of possible causes. And making an accurate diagnosis can be extremely difficult. In a scientific paper read to the Royal Society of Medicine in London recently a British surgeon who had analysed the diagnoses made on 416 children discovered that although a third were diagnosed as having appendicitis, in nearly half of the cases no diagnosis at all was ever made.

A completely comprehensive list of all the possible causes of abdominal pain would take up thousands of pages and be so long as to be quite useless. I have, however, compiled a list of some of the commonest causes of abdominal pain in children.

1 Appendicitis The appendix is a tube of intestine about the same size as its owner's little finger. It has no exit and is attached to the main intestinal route in much the same sort of way as a small cul-de-sac might be attached to a main road. Although various functions have been ascribed to the appendix it doesn't seem to have any real job to do as far as digesting food is concerned. Problems develop when pellets of food mistakenly find their way into the appendix, get stuck and obstruct the only entrance and exit to and from the appendix. That produces the inflammation and accompanying pain of appendicitis.

According to most of the classical textbooks used by doctors the appendix usually lies on the right hand side of the abdomen, just an inch or two above the right groin. The pain of appendicitis is usually said to start in the centre of the abdomen, round the umbilicus, and to move slowly down towards the right groin. Unfortunately for parents, doctors and children, the inflamed appendix does not always seem to know just what it is supposed to do. In practice just about any type of abdominal pain, with or without any other symptom, may indicate an appendix that needs removing.

The main risk with appendicitis is that the appendix can become so swollen and inflamed that it can burst, allowing pus to pour out into the abdominal cavity and producing a potentially dangerous generalised infection. The risk of an inflamed appendix perforating goes up as the hours go by. If an appendix stays inflamed for more than twenty-four hours then the risk can be considerable. If a swollen appendix bursts, pain temporarily disappears and a false sense of security may set in. Although perforation of the appendix is relatively rare in adults it is quite common in children. Between a third and a half of all children with appendicitis perforate before they receive treatment.

2 Constipation About one in ten of the children admitted to hospital with abdominal pain have nothing more than constipation. The pain develops as the muscular walls of the bowel struggle unsuccessfully to force hardened faeces along towards the intestinal exit. Constipation is discussed on page 88.

3 Mesenteric adenitis This condition is usually associated with a respiratory tract infection. The organism which causes the throat or chest infection, and which often produces swollen glands in the throat and neck, also has an effect on the lymph glands in the abdomen. The enlarged abdominal glands can then produce pain.

It is often difficult to make an accurate diagnosis when mesenteric adenitis is the cause of a child's pain. However, while a child with appendicitis will usually complain of a persistent pain a child with mesenteric adenitis will usually complain of a pain that comes and goes. And whereas the child with an inflamed appendix will usually lie very still the child with swollen abdominal glands will usually move around on the bed quite a good deal.

4 Pneumonia Some children with pneumonia do not have any marked chest signs but do have abdominal pain. However, even when there aren't any clear chest signs there will usually be an increase in the respiratory rate.

5 Cystitis Young children with urinary tract infections who have pain when they pass urine may well *seem* to have abdominal pains. If the infection spreads from the bladder back up towards the kidneys then the child may indeed have pains that are in his abdomen.

6 Gastroenteritis If a child has abdominal pain and severe diarrhoea then the chances are high that an infection of the intestinal tract is the cause. The infection will have probably been introduced in food and for this reason there will usually be others with the same symptoms – other members of the family, friends, school friends and so on. The pain tends to go away with each fresh bout of diarrhoea and to build up again just before the next bout. Although the pain itself can be quite severe there isn't usually very much tenderness in the abdomen.

If you push and press on the abdominal wall of a child with appendicitis then he'll probably cry or push you away with some passion. That sort of tenderness is rare with gastroenteritis.

7 Other physical causes Other disorders as varied as meningitis and diabetes can occasionally produce abdominal pains.

8 Stress and anxiety Although I have left 'stress' until the end it is perhaps one of the most important causes of abdominal pain in children. A remarkably high proportion of children who complain of physical pain have nothing obviously wrong with them when they are examined clinically and several large studies dealing with hundreds of young patients have shown that between a third and a half of all appendices removed are perfectly healthy. Subsequent studies, examining the owners of those healthy appendices, have shown that in many cases there is a strong history of stress, anxiety and pressure. Although it is difficult to prove a firm link between anxiety and abdominal pain the circumstantial evidence is powerful.

The evidence is particularly strong for the existence of a link between stress and strains and recurrent abdominal pains. These pains are usually situated in the centre of the abdomen, they are usually rather vague and they vary a lot. Classically these recurrent abdominal pains are associated with *specific* stresses and pressures. For example, the pains will start early in the morning and prevent a child going to school. Then, during the day, the pains will disappear. They'll reappear in the evening as the prospect of another day at school looms ahead.

9 Dietary indiscretions The child who eats an unripe apple or who gorges himself on too many pieces of cake will probably complain of an abdominal pain afterwards. Incidentally, it isn't the fact that the apple is unripe that causes the pain so much as the fact that the sourness of the apple prevents the child from chewing it properly. It's the chunks of apple in the stomach that cause the pain.

10 The unknown causes Most cases of abdominal pain will never be properly diagnosed. Don't feel too bad if you don't know what is causing your child's pain. Doctors know that they can only get a correct diagnosis about 50 per cent of the time. It's far more important that you should know what to do – and whether or not your child's pains need professional action.

11 Injury It's easy to forget injury as a possible cause of abdominal pain. The child who has received a blow to his abdomen could have suffered damage to his internal organs.

12 Peptic ulceration Although we usually associate peptic ulceration with business executives it is a condition which can develop in quite young children. If your child complains of an upper abdominal pain which seems to be related in some way to food then peptic ulceration is a possible diagnosis.

How do we make the diagnosis?
You should not try to make the diagnosis when your child has abdominal pain. Even trained medical specialists have difficulty in making a correct diagnosis more than half the time. The important question that you should try to answer is not 'What is wrong?' but 'Do we need the doctor?'

To answer these questions safely I suggest that you ask yourself the following questions:

1 Has the pain been present for more than a few hours?
2 Is the pain getting worse?
3 Has the pain developed since any blow or injury to the abdomen?
4 Has our child passed any red blood in or with his faeces?
5 Is the pain accompanied by pallor, sweating and/or breathlessness?
6 Is our child lying still to minimise the pain?
7 Is there a fever?
8 Is he breathing faster than usual?
9 Is there a fixed swelling in one or both groins?
10 Is there a painful or swollen scrotum?
11 Is he jaundiced?
12 Has he lost weight?
13 Has he suffered from persistent or recurrent diarrhoea or constipation?
14 Has he vomited any bright red or dark brown substance?
15 Do home remedies fail to relieve the pain?
16 Is he refusing to eat?

If the answer to any question is 'yes' then you need a doctor's advice. Now.

What can we do about it?

Once you've decided that your child does *not* need immediate medical attention for his abdominal pain then these are two things you must do.

First, you must observe him carefully in order to watch for any changes or deterioration in his condition.

Second, you must do all you can to make him as comfortable as possible. Home remedies such as simple painkillers and a good old-fashioned hot-water bottle will help a great deal. But comfort, sympathy, reassurance and tender loving care have an extremely important part to play. Mix sympathy with encouragement and pains will often disappear.

What will the doctor do?

Just as your major decision must be not 'What is wrong?' but 'Do we need to call the doctor?' so the doctor's most important decision must be not 'What is wrong?' but 'Does this patient need to be admitted to hospital?' It is far more important for him to decide whether or not surgical intervention is required than for him to attempt to make a firm and early diagnosis.

Once this decision has been made then naturally the next decisions will be governed by the making of a diagnosis. The action the doctor takes will depend on the nature of the problems.

Accidents

What are they?

Very few accidents are entirely inexplicable or completely unavoidable. When children seem to be accident-prone there is usually a reason. In order to minimise the number of accidents your child has you must first understand what risks exist and precisely how accidents develop.

How common are they?

Accidents are the commonest cause of death in all children over the age of 1 year. The top ten causes of accidental death are:

1 Being hit by a motor vehicle while walking or while riding a bicycle.
2 Drowning.
3 Being involved in a road traffic accident as a car passenger.

4 Fire.

5 Falling.

6 Suffocation.

7 Choking.

8 Poisoning.

9 Electrical problems.

10 Explosions.

Accidents in these categories cause more deaths among children than pneumonia, meningitis, cancer, heart disease and congenital problems put together. Moreover, while the number of children dying from each of these medical disorders is falling annually the number of children dying from accidents is not changing.

At what age are children most vulnerable to accidents?

Babies under the age of 1 year are usually relatively immobile and therefore not as much at risk as their older brothers and sisters. When babies do get hurt it is usually because they have been dropped, laid down carelessly or injured because of carelessness on the part of some older person.

Over the age of 1 year all children are vulnerable to accidents. Accidents are the major cause of death and serious illness in all people between the ages of 1 year old and the mid-thirties!

Is it true that some children are just naturally clumsy or accident-prone?

Parents whose children are almost permanently decorated with pieces of sticking plaster or who are such regular customers of the local hospital emergency department that they are invariably greeted by their Christian names will usually claim that their children are simply accident-prone. There are even many learned papers in the medical journals in which respected members of the medical profession have discussed the problem of 'accident-proneness'.

I'm afraid, however, that I don't believe that there is any such thing as accident-proneness. When children repeatedly have accidents then there are usually reasons for it. Accidents are not 'accidental' at all, they don't occur because of completely unforeseen circumstances. They occur because someone, some-where has been careless or ignorant or because of some physical disability.

Why do accidents happen?

1 Because of poor sight or hearing Children who are not able to see or hear clearly will obviously be more 'prone' to accidental injury. If a child's visual or hearing disability has not been identified or corrected then the appropriate treatment may make a startling difference to the family's consumption of antiseptic fluid and sticking plaster.

2 Because of a brain disorder Very rarely clumsy children turn out to have neurological problems. A child who is unable to direct and control his muscles accurately will be in danger of having many accidents.

3 Because of epilepsy When children have minor seizures their temporary loss of consciousness may go unnoticed except for the fact that they seem to be 'accident-prone'.

4 Because of boredom The child who is bored will allow his concentration to lapse. This is particularly likely to be a problem with intelligent children.

5 Because of simple carelessness It's astonishing just how many so-called accidents are a result of thoughtlessness or stupidity either on the part of the child or a parent. If a child rides a bicycle straight out on to a main road and is hit by a passing car then the incident can hardly be described as an accident. If a small child takes an overdose of pretty coloured pills because a bottle of tablets has been left on the kitchen table then the overdose can hardly be called an accident.

6 Stress and anxiety The child who is worrying about school exams, his prowess on the sports field or his relationship with his parents will be unable to concentrate on what he is doing. He'll be far more likely to have repeated accidents.

7 Drugs and medicines Many modern drugs (even those which are bought over the counter without a prescription) can cause drowsiness. A child who has been given large quantities of cough medicine and who is half asleep all the time will be 'accident-prone.'

8 Hormones It is now well established that many girls are more likely to have accidents just before they have a period than at any other time. The week before a period starts seems to be the danger time for the majority of sufferers with the final days being the most dangerous. The hormonal changes which occur as a period approaches make girls more irritable, aggressive and depressed and less able to concentrate. There is also a change in a girl's capacity to co-ordinate muscle activity. Hormone changes can cause clumsiness and clumsiness causes accidents. (See the section on menstrual problems, page 178.)

How can we reduce the risk of our child having an accident?
1 If your child has repeated accidents do make sure that there is no physical explanation. If you are uncertain about this visit your doctor and ask him to check your child to exclude the possibility of a sight or hearing problem or a neurological disorder of some kind.
2 Do be aware of the risks to children which may vary very much from the risks which face adults. You can't eradicate all risks but you can minimise your child's exposure to hazard.
3 Road accidents are a common cause of death and serious injury in children of all ages. Even babies and children under the age of 1 year are at risk when travelling in motor vehicles. Follow these rules to avoid excessive risk:

(a) Do not allow children to travel on their parent's lap in the front passenger seat of motor cars.
(b) Children travelling in motor cars should use seat belts. Smaller children and babies should travel in special seats fitted with appropriate restraint systems.
(c) Teach your child that roads are dangerous places. Do not allow him to play on roads where cars pass by – even if the traffic is light.
(d) Teach your child the basic rules of road safety as early as you can.
(e) Do not allow a child to ride a bicycle on public roads until he has mastered his machine and the elementary rules of safe riding.
(f) Remember that children usually find it difficult to judge the road speed of vehicles. Do not allow a child to cross major roads by himself until he has learnt how to do so safely.

(g) Put child-proof locks on rear car doors if they aren't already fitted.

(h) If your child has a bicycle make sure that it is kept in good working condition with tyres, lights and brakes checked regularly.

4 Every year thousands of children are poisoned. Many die and many more suffer agonies. Poisoning is never really accidental. If you obey the following rules you should be able to minimise the risk of your child becoming just another sad poisoning statistic.

(a) Child-resistant containers may be a nuisance but they do provide some protection should a child manage to get hold of a pill bottle. If you have a child in your home insist on your pills being dispensed in child-proof containers.

(b) Pills of all kinds should be kept in medicine cabinets which need to be locked and out of reach. Even medicines bought over the counter need to be locked out of reach. Although a small dose of a drug obtained without a prescription may be safe enough a large dose may still be fatal.

(c) When your child visits an older relative make sure that there aren't any pills or pill containers lying around. Older people aren't always used to having inquisitive children around.

(d) Never pour poisons out of their proper containers into old lemonade bottles. Every year children who think they're drinking something thirst-quenching die because they've taken a mouthful of bleach or weedkiller.

(e) Teach your children the dangers of household products and let them see that you take those dangers seriously. You don't have to instill terror – caution and respect will do.

(f) Throw away any unwanted medicines or potential poisons.

(g) Never encourage children to take medicines by telling them that they taste good or by pretending that they are sweets.

(h) Keep all household products that can be dangerous in the same place. If possible keep that cupboard locked.

(i) If you're interrupted by the telephone or doorbell while working with a potentially dangerous substance take it with you or fasten the container before leaving it. Many children have been poisoned while mother chatters to a friend on the telephone.

(j) If a label on a container comes off replace the label straight away. If you're not sure what is in the container then throw the contents away.

(k) If you're carrying freshly cleaned clothes in your car travel with the windows open wide. The fumes from the cleaning fluids can be dangerous.

(l) Make sure that you know what to do in a poisoning emergency (see page 5).

5 Your home can be a death trap unless you take care to minimise the risk of an accident taking place.

(a) If you have an open fire make sure that you use a fire guard.

(b) Keep plugs in sockets when children are playing in a room.

(c) If you live high up make sure that you don't allow children to play near windows which aren't equipped with safety catches.

(d) Make sure that damaged or worn electrical wiring is replaced.

(e) Never leave plastic bags of any shape or size lying around.

(f) Don't put mirrors on the chimney breast above a fire of any kind. Small children (particularly girls in party dresses) are often tempted to stand too close to admire themselves. The results can be horrifying.

(g) Keep all sharp objects (scissors, knives and so on) well out of reach. Plastic scissors are fine for cutting paper but won't cut skin.

(h) Don't leave children alone with oil or paraffin heaters.

(i) Don't let children get into bed with electric blankets still plugged in.

(j) Small children shouldn't be given small toys to play with. Nor should they be given toys which can be taken apart and turned into smaller pieces.

(k) Stair carpets should be well fixed. When there are very young children around a safety gate should be fixed at the top and bottom of the stairs.

(l) Don't have loose rugs on polished floors.

6 Burns and scalds are common among children. They can be avoided.

(a) Never put saucepans on a stove in such a way that the handles stick out. Children often pull hot liquids down over themselves.

(b) Don't leave a container with anything hot in it near the edge of a table.

(c) Put matches and lighters out of reach.

(d) Don't let children play with cookers or stoves.

(e) Hot tap water is a common source of burns among children. Because children frequently climb into baths filled with water that is too hot the burns are often over large areas of skin. Hot water shouldn't be heated beyond 50° centigrade (120°F).

7 Gardens and playgrounds can be hazardous too. You can limit the hazard by following these rules.

(a) If you have any playground equipment (such as a slide, swing and so on) make sure that it is kept in good working condition. If possible install equipment in such a way that a child who falls off will fall on to grass or sand. (The equipment itself should, of course, be firmly anchored to a solid base.) Small children should be supervised on swings.

(b) Keep swimming pools, paddling pools and ornamental ponds covered when no adults are around.

(c) Children should be taught to recognise dangerous bushes and plants and taught never to eat berries they cannot identify with absolute certainty.

(d) Children should be taught to regard all wild mushrooms as potentially toxic.

(e) Never let children play with bonfires and never burn household refuse on bonfires when children are around. Old chairs and painted furniture can give off dangerous fumes.

(g) Don't let children play on grass that has been fouled by animals.

(h) If your garden leads out on to a road make sure that your gate fastens firmly and is kept fastened.

(i) If you have used a weedkiller on the garden read the instructions carefully and keep your child away for the appropriate period of time.

(j) Don't let children try athletic tricks that they have seen on television until they have been properly trained. Children who try to emulate highly successful high jumpers and pole vaulters can easily have nasty falls.

Acne

What is it?
Acne affects older children and teenagers. Spots on the face, neck and back sometimes become red and infected.

What causes it?
Deep inside the skin there are a number of special cells and glands. The sebaceous glands, which are usually attached to hair follicles, produce a substance called sebum which is itself a mixture of fatty acids, cholesterol, waxes and broken-down cells. The sebaceous glands have a most important function; they produce what is effectively an automatic emollient designed to protect the skin from becoming too dry. An absence of sebum means that the skin becomes dry and scaly. When there is too much sebum the skin becomes greasy and oily to the touch.

The production of sebum is increased by a number of factors but one of the most important is the rise in sex hormones which occurs in the years of puberty. In men the hormone is the one which is responsible for the development of the male patterns of hair growth and for the development of a deep voice and other secondary sexual characteristics. In girls the hormone concerned is the one which helps to trigger menstrual flow. It is this relationship between the relatively sudden increase in the availability of sex hormone and the consequent increase in the amount of sebum secreted which explains the high incidence of greasy skin among teenagers.

In addition to changes in the hormone level (and subsequent changes in the amount of sebum being secreted) there are other changes occurring at about this time. In particular, the outer horny layer of the skin tends to get thicker.

Problems arise and acne develops if the ducts through which the sebum travels from the sebaceous glands to the skin's surface become blocked. Dead skin cells are the commonest type of blockage. When these have been stuck for a while in a duct they turn black – producing blackheads. Later they may become infected, producing red, swollen acne spots.

Is it infectious?
Acne is not infectious in the way that diseases such as measles and chickenpox are infectious. You aren't likely to catch it from

another sufferer. But the so-called blackheads do sometimes become infected.

Does diet make acne worse?
It used to be said that eating chocolates and fatty foods made acne worse. It is now generally accepted that there is no real relationship between diet and acne.

What can we do about it?
There is still a good deal of confusion about what makes acne worse and what is likely to make it better. But it is fairly well agreed that one of the most important things to do is to keep the pores clear of sebum and dead cells. If the pores are kept clear and there are no blackheads then there will be no acne spots.

The simplest way to keep the pores clear is to wash the skin regularly with a rather rough abrasive of some kind. It does not matter much whether this is a special cleansing paste, a special cleansing sponge, a fairly soft brush, an electric face cleanser or just a rough face cloth. Some beauty editors suggest using almonds ground in milk, strawberries or orange peel – all these would effectively act as simple abrasives.

Sometimes these simple abrasives don't keep the pores cleaned out thoroughly enough. When this is the problem then a substance called a keratolytic can be used. The keratolytics most commonly used are resorcinol, salicylic acid and benoxyl peroxide, and these are available singly or in combination in a number of products. Whatever you choose a keratolytic works by unblocking the pores and cleaning out the blackheads.

Young people with acne spots always want to squeeze them to get rid of them quicker. Parents sometimes tell them not to and warn that squeezing spots simply makes them worse. If an uninfected blackhead can be removed then it is probably better to remove it although it is important to ensure that the skin of the face and hands is washed first. Fingernails, if used with care, are probably just as safe and effective as comedo expressors sold by chemists. Infected spots should never be squeezed since by doing so you can spread the infection and make things worse.

It is a good idea to persuade children with spotty skin to get as much sunshine as possible since ultraviolet light encourages skin peeling and that should help unblock ducts. Keeping hair short may also help since greasy skin is often accompanied by greasy hair – the combination tends to make everything worse.

Make-up can contribute to the problem. Thick foundations, creams, pastes, powders and so on block pores and make the development of spots much more likely and the perpetuation of existing spots almost certain. Young girls with a susceptibility to acne should, therefore, be wary of using make-up at all. When they *do* use make-up they should certainly be careful to remove it all afterwards.

Finally, it is important to offer acne sufferers as much help and reassurance as possible. Don't say 'you'll grow out of it' because the acne sufferer is usually worried about 'now', not 'tomorrow'.

What about proprietary products for acne?

Acne is a problem which affects millions of young people for months or even years at a time. There are, therefore, a number of companies involved in the manufacture and sale of special remedies for the prevention and treatment of acne.

Some of these products are said to open and close the skin pores and to control the formation of blackheads. Others are said to contain antiseptics which will clear away spots in days. There are even products sold for their value in clearing away from the blood those impurities which lead to the development of acne. In my view most of these products are rubbish.

When do we need to see the doctor?

Although acne is never a dangerous disease it can be very worrying. The mental damage can far outweigh the physical damage that is done. For this reason I suggest that if spots cannot be controlled to the patient's satisfaction then it is a good idea to see a doctor. Your family doctor may then refer the young patient to a skin specialist. It is always worthwhile referring the child to a doctor when the spots are obviously infected.

What will the doctor do?

If the acne spots are badly infected then your doctor may prescribe an antibiotic such as tetracycline or a sulphonamide. These drugs need to be taken by mouth. Antibiotics won't stop spots being formed but they will help clear away superficial signs of infection.

To clear out blocked pores doctors sometimes prescribe powerful keratolytics but they also prescribe chemical or mechanical abrasive procedures when things are really bad. These remedies are unlikely to be needed for simple teenage acne.

Allergy reactions

What are they?
The human body has a sophisticated series of internal defence mechanisms designed to help provide protection against a vast variety of different threats. One of the most important protective systems is the body's immunological defences. It is the immunological system which enables the human body to protect itself against infections.

Efficient as it is, however, the human immunological system will sometimes overreact to foreign substances; switching on special defence systems which aren't needed and producing uncomfortable and sometimes violent symptoms which are in practice more of a threat than the cause of the response!

What causes them?
Allergy reactions can develop to foreign substances which enter the body through the nose or through the mouth or which simply come into contact with the skin. A vast variety of different substances can cause allergy reactions. It is probably true to say that there is no substance in the world to which some individual has not at some time or another developed an allergy reaction. Pollens, dust, foods and animals are perhaps the commonest causes of reactions.

About one in five of all children have an allergy reaction of some kind and whether or not a particular child develops an allergy to a particular substance depends largely on genetic factors. (It is now clear that children inherit a susceptibility to allergy reactions.)

The type of allergy reaction a child has depends on a number of different factors but it is important to remember that one child may suffer from one, two or even more different allergies.

What types of allergy reaction exist?
Below I have listed some of the commonest different types of allergy reactions.

1 Asthma Children who develop asthma are usually allergic to grass pollen, dust or animals. Asthma is one of the most serious allergy diseases since it can lead to great physical distress. It is discussed at greater length on page 33.

2 Eczema Eczema commonly occurs because of an allergy reaction which develops in the skin. Eczema in children seems to be commonly associated with foodstuffs that have been eaten. Excluding the appropriate substance from the diet usually solves the problem. See page 120.

3 Allergic rhinitis This is one of the commonest forms of allergy reactions. Many children who seem to suffer permanently from colds do in fact suffer from allergic rhinitis. A child who seems to suffer from a permanent runny nose, congestion, catarrh and sneezing should be considered a possible sufferer from allergic rhinitis.

4 Hay fever When a child is allergic to a substance which appears on the scene seasonally the symptoms will obviously appear seasonally too. Hay fever is perhaps the best example of a seasonal allergy. See page 148.

5 Migraine There is a good deal of evidence to suggest that migraine headaches and other symptoms are caused by allergy reactions. Specific foods such as chocolate, broad beans, red wine and bananas have been identified as causing migraine. See page 180.

This list is very limited. Many other disorders are known to be caused by allergy reactions to different substances. Gastro-intestinal colic and arthritis are just two diseases sometimes said to be caused by an allergy reaction. Otitis media and conjunctivitis are two disorders which may be commoner in children who suffer from allergic rhinitis and hay fever respectively.

How do we make the diagnosis?

Some allergy reactions are easy to spot. If a child suddenly starts to sneeze and complain of itchy eyes in the pollen season then it isn't too difficult to come up with a diagnosis of hay fever. If a child develops an angry-looking skin rash every time she uses a certain brand of soap then it doesn't take a diagnostic wizard to jump to the conclusion that there may be an allergy reaction at the root of the problem!

Some types of food allergy are fairly easy to spot too. If a child suddenly becomes ill and acquires a red, blotchy, itchy skin rash after eating a portion of strawberries or crab meat then it can safely be assumed that an allergy reaction has been produced.

The symptoms may not always be this obvious, however, and a child who has a food allergy may complain of symptoms which seem superficially unrelated to food. Vomiting, diarrhoea, stomach pains, eczema, asthma and allergic rhinitis are all disorders which can occur as a result of a food allergy.

What can we do about it?

1 If there is a family history of allergies of any kind (asthma, eczema, hay fever or whatever) then mother should consider breast feeding exclusively for six months. This will ensure that the baby is protected by his mother's own immunological system. It will also mean that the baby will not be exposed to the foreign substances which are present in cows' milk and which can easily produce an allergy reaction. It is important to ensure that only breast milk is taken since even small quantities of cows milk can trigger an allergic reaction.

2 If there is a clearly defined allergen of any kind then all possible attempts should be made to avoid contact with that allergen. If a child develops asthma when he has been in contact with cat fur then the obvious solution is to avoid cats. If a child has an allergy reaction every time he eats a particulr type of food then the obvious answer is to avoid that particular type of food.

3 Stress and pressure of all kind exacerbate allergy reactions. Avoiding excess stress helps reduce allergy symptoms (see page 288).

When to see the doctor

If your child has clear symptoms of an allergy problem or you think that his symptoms could be caused by an allergy reaction of some kind and your attempts to deal with the symptoms have been unsuccessful then you should seek medical advice.

What will the doctor do?

His first job will usually be to try and identify the nature of the allergen. If the history taking does not produce any useful evidence then this can be done by injecting minute amounts of all the possible allergens into the skin and then looking for signs of an allergy rection. Once the allergen has been identified then it will sometimes be possible to prepare a special desensitising course of injections.

A series of injections are planned so that the patient can be given a steadily increasing dose of the allergen concerned. His body will then slowly acquire properly coordinated immunological defences.

Alternatively the doctor may rely on antihistamines to provide symptomatic relief. These drugs effectively block the development of allergy symptoms.

Anorexia nervosa

What is it?
Although this extremely well publicised disease usually affects girls and young women it can also affect boys and men. The patient with anorexia nervosa refuses to eat, loses weight and gradually becomes thinner and thinner. If left untreated the patient may eventually starve herself to death. Although it has recently been the study of much public discussion anorexia nervosa has in fact been described in the medical journals for several centuries now.

What causes it?
Paediatricians and psychiatrists, psychologists and physicians are all continually arguing about precisely what produces anorexia nervosa. It is thought by one group that anorexia is simply a consequence of our society's overemphasis on the slim figure. Those who favour this theory are able to produce a good deal of evidence in support of their contention. They can, for example, point out that in one large Scandinavian survey researchers found that dieting was commonplace even among girls of normal weight. They can also point to an American study which showed that of 1000 high school teenagers 50 per cent considered themselves to be overweight whereas in fact only 25 per cent were. All the studies which have been done seem to show that it is mainly girls who worry about their weight. The general lack of interest among boys in their shape and weight is said to explain

the fact that anorexia nervosa is far commoner among girls than among boys.

So strong do some researchers feel is the link between what can perhaps best be described as 'social dieting' and anorexia nervosa that they sometimes claim that anorexia nervosa may indeed not be a separate disease at all, but simply an extreme type of dieting behaviour.

In contrast, however, there are also a number of clinicians who claim that anorexia nervosa is a consequence of some sort of psychological conflict, either within the sufferer's own mind or between the sufferer and her family. The studies quoted by this group of clinicians show that it is when parents expect too much of their children that anorexia nervosa is most likely to result. Pressure at school, pressure from contemporaries or pressure from relatives can all have a tremendous effect on potential sufferers from this disorder. Those who favour this theory point out that sufferers from anorexia nervosa are usually model children, always keen to please and do well.

Psychoanalysts have argued that the refusal of food is an expression of sexual conflict, a rejection of mother, a fear of oral impregnation by father, a rejection of adolescence and its accompanying sexual maturity or a desire to preserve the joys of childhood. Others have claimed that anorexia nervosa is a result of an obsessional desire to avoid food, a consequence of a deep feeling of depression or a result of a preoccupation with academic work. It has also been said that the mothers of children with anorexia nervosa are usually overprotective.

My own view is that anorexia nervosa is probably a single set of symptoms produced by a whole range of different factors. I suspect that there is some truth in the suggestion that pressure on children to succeed may produce anorexia nervosa, particularly when the pressure is applied at the time when the child is having to cope with the problems of puberty. But I also very strongly suspect that anorexia nervosa is often produced or made worse by our society's obsession with weight control.

How do we make the diagnosis?

Since normal appetite loss is rarely of any real significance (whereas anorexia nervosa always needs to be regarded seriously) it is obviously important to be able to differentiate between the two.

I have prepared below a list of the salient features of anorexia nervosa.

1 The patient will not only have a poor appetite but she may also show disgust at the very prospect of eating. Paradoxically she may also be preoccupied with food and may spend much of her time buying and cooking food for others.

2 The patient suffering from anorexia nervosa will invariably lose a good deal of weight. It is not uncommon for weight loss to be measured in stones rather than pounds.

3 Girls and boys who suffer from anorexia nervosa are usually overactive, particularly at night when they invariably find it difficult to get to sleep.

4 Girls who suffer from anorexia nervosa do not normally have any menstrual periods. Sexual development is usually arrested.

I believe that any parents who feel that their child has symptoms which fit into these categories should think of anorexia nervosa as a possible diagnosis. It is interesting to note, by the way, that many of the individuals who develop anorexia nervosa were at one time in their lives quite plump. It is this dramatic change from being overweight to being dramatically under-weight that has probably helped many doctors come to the conclusion that there is a link between anorexia nervosa and overenthusiastic dieting.

What can we do about it?

Anorexia nervosa, whatever its cause may be, can kill. It is important to recognise that it is an illness that needs to be taken seriously. Parents should be aware that sufferers from anorexia nervosa are often reluctant to accept the fact that they need medical attention, they are often reluctant to accept that anything they do is abnormal and despite the fact that they look emaciated they may still feel grossly overweight. In an attempt to deal with the concern of others, victims of this disorder will frequently try to disguise the fact that they are not eating and may, for example, hide food which they pretend to have eaten.

The first thing to be done is to persuade the patient who has anorexia nervosa that she needs help. Although the assistance of the patient's family is vital there is little doubt that the disorder requires professional help. I strongly suggest that whenever the disorder is suspected professional help be obtained just as soon as possible. Treatment is more difficult when the diagnosis is delayed – both because the weight loss may have become critical and because the psychological factors may have deteriorated.

What will the doctor do?
Since the causes of anorexia nervosa are still disputed by doctors it is hardly surprising that different doctors offer different types of treatment.

The first thing most doctors will do is to rule out any possibility that the weight loss may have been caused by any other physical or mental abnormality.

Next, an attempt will be made to help the patient regain the weight that she has lost. Different doctors use different approaches but basically the aim of the doctor who is looking after a patient with anorexia nervosa will be to build up a good relationship and to use that relationship as the basis for whatever form of psychological treatment is considered most appropriate.

Anxiety

What is it?
We all feel anxious, worried or nervous at some time or other and children are no different from adults in this respect. Under normal circumstances anxiety can be regarded as a fairly acceptable human emotion. Life without anxiety would be just as incomplete as life without happiness.

However, there are times when anxiety becomes an over-dominant emotion and develops out of all proportion. When this occurs the anxiety may cause any one of a number of physical and mental symptoms.

What causes it?
There are thousands of different causes of anxiety. Potentially anxious individuals will often worry about things which may seem irrational or unimportant. Children are no more and no less likely to worry about imaginary insults or threats than adults and the causes of anxiety are not always entirely rational.

One of the commonest causes of anxiety among young children is excessive pressure applied either by parents or by school-teachers. Young boys and girls are these days often encouraged to stay at school for as long as possible and to acquire as many certificates and diplomas as they possibly can. There are good reasons for this but it is nevertheless a fact that this type of stress frequently causes anxiety. It is equally true to say that the pressure on a child to succeed in sporting activities is also a very real cause of anxiety. Young swimmers, gymnasts, athletes, footballers and all who show any hint of real talent are often put under almost intolerable pressure while even the less than talented are encouraged to worry about team success, league positions, trophies and so on. These pressures and stresses are, within certain limits, good for all children. However, while a few children may be able to cope comfortably with tremendous pressures others will be far more susceptible. They will worry about failure and about being unable to satisfy the demands and expectations of those whom they regard with love and respect.

How can we tell if our child is suffering from anxiety?

Stress and anxiety produce a wide range of physical and mental symptoms. The overanxious child may have difficulty in getting to sleep, he may be irritable and unable to concentrate effectively, he may seem to cry more than usual and he may have a poor memory. He may be unable to finish things he's started, he may be impulsive and he may also seem intolerant and unable to relax.

Among the physical problems made worse by anxiety are skin disorders such as eczema and dermatitis, chest problems such as asthma, bowel disorders such as constipation and diarrhoea and miscellaneous stomach aches. Headaches are another common problem. Many tics and habits such as thumb sucking and nail biting are common symptoms of anxiety.

These symptoms sometimes occur in such a way that it is possible to recognise a direct association between the symptoms produced by anxiety and the cause. For example, the child who has a stomach ache every Monday morning or who has difficulty in getting to sleep every Sunday night is probably worried about going to school.

Very occasionally children, like adults, may suffer from anxiety attacks. When this happens the child will usually panic, breathe rapidly and shallowly and be obviously very alarmed. Panic attacks are best dealt with by trying to calm the child and by encouraging him to take slow deep breaths. If this doesn't work a doctor's advice must be sought.

What can we do about it?
It is obviously best to treat any type of anxiety or any anxiety-induced problem by attending to the cause of the anxiety rather than by simply dealing with the symptoms. To deal only with the symptom is like repapering a damp patch in the bedroom instead of dealing with the hole in the roof that is causing it. The child who feels that he is expected to perform to high standards in either academic or sporting fields will benefit most from reassurance and encouragement. He needs to be assured that those whom he loves and respects will not think any the less of him, or love him any less, should he fail to live up to the standards he thinks they expect. This is an important point because sometimes parents are not aware of the fact that their children feel under pressure to do well.

When do we need to see a doctor?
If a child has an acute anxiety attack it is usually wise to see a doctor for a little general advice. If a child seems to be suffering from symptoms which you suspect are caused by stress but for which you can find no explanation it will also be worth seeking medical advice. When anxiety symptoms relate specifically to particular fears it is worthwhile seeking medical advice at an early stage since otherwise it is possible for simple fears to grow into fully-fledged phobias (see page 204).

Appetite loss (anorexia)

What is it?
The human body has an automatic appetite control centre which is designed to regulate the owner's intake of food. A study that was published in the *American Journal of Diseases of Children* showed that when infants just a few months old were allowed to choose what they ate from a range of simple, natural foods they automatically selected diets which contained a perfect balance of essential nutrients. Not only did they carefully organise their eating habits to ensure that they ate the right types of food but they also automatically limited their *total* intake of food. Another scientific study showed that young children will automatically choose foods that enable them to avoid digestive upsets such as constipation and diarrhoea. A third study showed that individuals

adapt their eating habits according to the outside temperature.

These and other pieces of research all show fairly conclusively that the appetite control centre has a great influence over the body's intake of food. Although we do know that many of us deliberately overrule our own appetite control mechanisms (see the section on obesity, page 190) we still don't really know how the centre is stimulated. Research has shown that appetite tends to be increased by the sight of food and by the lowering of the blood sugar level but no one yet knows precisely why and how the appetite control centre is stimulated to reduce the appetite.

What causes it?

Although we may not know too much about the pathways through which appetite loss is organised we do know a considerable amount about what sort of conditions can cause appetite loss. It is well known, for example, that the commonest cause of apetite loss is illness. Most children who are ill, even though they may only have some relatively minor infectious disorder, will be less interested in food than they would otherwise have been.

Another common, and often very worrying cause of appetite loss is the condition known as negativism. Young children commonly go through a stage during which they deliberately oppose all their parents' wishes. This is merely a manifestation of ego development but it is obviously extremely worrying since the child involved is likely to oppose all his parents' most enthusiastic expectations. The child who isn't ill but who will not eat at all will soon find that he can manipulate his parents very effectively by continuing his hunger strike. The more his parents bribe or threaten him the more he is likely to hold out. There is a real risk with this common condition that if the parents respond too dramatically and punish their child every time he fails to eat then the child will eventually associate food and fear. That association can lead to a long-term reduction in appetite.

Far less serious but probably just as common is the type of appetite loss which results from an excessive consumption of between-meal snacks. The child who incessantly chews sweets and chocolate is unlikely to have much room left for his main meals.

The other main type of appetite loss that I haven't mentioned is, of course, the condition known as anorexia nervosa in which the

victim, usually but not always a young girl, will refuse food so
steadfastly that she may eventually starve herself to death. I have
described this condition and the symptoms and signs which
characterise it, on page 25.

Finally, I must point out that in many instances parents worry
that their children aren't eating enough when in fact their own
expectations are far too high. Put in print it looks a remarkably
silly thing to say but small children do need less food than large
children.

What can we do about it?

There are no magic 'tonics' which will influence a child's appetite.
Nor, indeed, is there any need for any such mysterious appetite
stimulants. It is equally important to remember that attempts to
force a child to eat will almost always end in failure.

The first thing that must be done is for you to take some
decision about whether or not your child really does have a poor
appetite and, if so, exactly what is causing the loss of appetite. If
your child has an infectious disease, for example, then appetite
loss is almost inevitable. This is nothing to worry about since no
child is going to starve as a result of a diminished appetite for a
few days. It is, however, important to ensure that fluid intake is
maintained since fluid loss is much more likely to produce a
dramatic effect. If your child is passing less urine than usual then
this is an important sign that he is drinking too little.

To encourage his appetite try and make sure that you present
food as attractively as possible. Try to select foods that you know
are favourites and be careful not to put too much food on his
plate. The child with a poor appetite who is presented with a
massive plateful of food probably won't eat anything at all
because he'll be disheartened and dispirited by the sight of so
much food. The child who has a poor appetite and is offered a
small portion of food may well eat that and then ask for more.
Remember too that children don't necessarily have to eat at
mealtimes and although it may be inconvenient to have to
prepare food to order it is probably sensible to do so if you're
trying to encourage your child's appetite.

If your child's appetite loss doesn't seem to be related to a
specific illness, or if you feel that there is any associated weight
loss, then you should probably ask for some medical guidance.
There isn't likely to be much that your doctor can do apart from

offer reassurance but he may be able to help you understand precisely why your child's appetite seems to have disappeared. It may be that you've been too enthusiastic about food and that your child is simply rebelling against you.

Before finishing this section I should just mention the problem of food fads. These are usually the result of a child's attempts to manipulate his parents rather than the result of a genuine inability to eat a particular type of food. Don't overreact when your child objects to certain types of food. The parent who allows a battle of wills to develop over one particular type of food is quite likely to find himself fighting a losing battle. A little gentle encouragement at an early stage is far better than a lot of heavy pressure later on when the fad has become well established.

When should we see the doctor?

If your child's appetite loss has continued for more than five days, is not the obvious result of a disorder which is now resolving, or is accompanied by a weight loss of more than a couple of pounds, then you should seek medical advice.

Asthma

What is it?

Asthma is one of the commonest chronic childhood illnesses and almost certainly the subject of more myths and misconceptions than any other childhood illness.

Asthma develops because the tubes which carry air into the lungs become obstructed. Some inborn factor means that the muscles which surround the air passages react too rapidly and too easily while the lining inside the passageways has a tendency to swell. Triggered by some external factors (which I'll describe in a moment) the linings swell and the muscular walls contract. There is then a narrowing of the airways.

How do we make the diagnosis?

The basic signs and symptoms which identify the asthma sufferer are:

1 Wheezing which is usually more obvious on breathing out.
2 Breathlessness – most children with asthma complain that they cannot get enough air into their chests.

3 Coughing.

4 These three symptoms come and go – occasionally disappearing altogether. They are sometimes present individually and sometimes together.

What causes it?

In most cases childhood asthma is caused by the child being allergic to something with which he has been in contact. There would be no point at all in my trying to produce a comprehensive list of the things to which sufferers can be allergic because the list would be virtually endless – it's perhaps enough to say that grasses, pollen, house dust and cat fur are among the commonest allergens.

When asthma is produced in this way the body's reaction is much the same as it is to any other allergen. If a child's arm comes into contact with some substance to which the child is allergic then the skin of the arm will become red and swollen. The mechanism may be slightly different but in allergic asthma what happens is that the passageways within the lungs react to an allergen which has been breathed in either through the nose or the mouth.The swollen, aggravated passageways impede the passage of air and cause the breathlessness and wheezing that are such significant symptoms with asthma.

If the characteristic wheezing obviously occurs whenever the child is in contact with some particular object then it isn't too difficult to deduce the nature of the allergy. But in the majority of cases things aren't that easy. Indeed, it may be extremely difficult to try and isolate the link between the wheezing and whatever the causative factor is.

Sometimes it is possible to identify the cause of the allergy by a series of skin tests. When this has been done it may then be possible to give the child a series of desensitising injections which work in much the same sort of way as a vaccination programme.

So far I've only mentioned allergy as a possible cause of childhood asthma. It is, however, important to remember that there are other possible causes. Infections can make wheezing much worse if they affect the respiratory system and can produce a type of asthma in some children. This link between asthma and infection means that any asthmatic child who gets a cold should be treated with perhaps a little more care than average. He may need to be seen by a doctor at a rather earlier stage than the non-asthmatic child and he may need to be given a prophylactic antibiotic if it is known that mild chest infections invariably lead to a worsening of the situation.

The quality of the air a child is breathing can also have an effect on his susceptibility to asthma. It is now well known that cold air, very dry air, air polluted by cigarette smoke and air heated by gas or polluted by cooking smells can all make asthma worse.

The other really important point to remember is that asthma can be made much worse by emotional upsets and worry of all kinds. If an asthma sufferer seems to be wheezing a good deal for no apparent reason it may well be anxiety which is making things worse.

Is it infectious?
No.

Who gets it? Is our child likely to get asthma?
Asthma can be inherited and if one or both parents suffered from asthma or suffer from asthma then a child has about a one in ten chance of getting the disease. It doesn't seem to make any difference to the child's chances of getting asthma whether one or both parents were sufferers. Where there is no family history of asthma then about one in twenty children are affected. Boys seem slightly more likely to suffer from asthma than girls and the first symptoms usually begin before the child reaches the age of 5 years.

What is the outlook?
Three out of four childhood sufferers from asthma will grow out of the disease. Out of all the children who have asthma only one in four will have it as an adult.

What can we do about it?
The first and perhaps most useful piece of advice I can give is to recommend that you try and ignore all the 'good' advice and 'warnings' which you are offered by well-meaning friends and relatives. Asthma is a disorder which needs to be taken seriously but it is a condition which seems to bring out the worst in well-meaning friends and relatives.

One of the most common things that parents are told is that all children who have asthma will also get eczema. (This advice is always given the other way round as well, of course, and mothers whose children have eczema will always be told that asthma will follow in due course.) It is true that there is a relationship between these two disorders in that both can be produced by allergy reactions. But it is not true that every child with asthma will get eczema any more than it is true that every child with eczema will automatically develop asthma.

If your child does have an allergic asthma and you are lucky enough to be able to find out just what causes the wheezing then it is not difficult to see how best you can help your child! But if you haven't been able to find out exactly which allergens are responsible it may not be quite so easy to solve the problem.

When that is the case and the cause of the asthma has remained something of a mystery then it is usually a good idea to use cotton or nylon bed linen instead of wool, to avoid feather pillows and to be particularly careful to clear away all dust. I mention this last point with some trepidation because I realise that most of my readers will throw up their arms in horror and dismay at the unwritten suggestion that they might allow dust to remain in their homes.

The fact is, however, that dust can gather on tops of wardrobes and in the far corners of closets and that this dust can initiate asthma attacks in some children.

The question of what to do about pets is a difficult one. If a child can be shown to have a definite allergy to a particular pet then a decision has to be taken: whether to upset the child by taking the pet away or whether to allow the pet to remain and to put up with the resultant asthma. There is no simple answer to that dilemma. As a general rule it is probably best to avoid the problem as far as possible by avoiding pets if a child is asthmatic. If a family pet is too well loved to be given away then it is probably best to resist the temptation to replace that pet when it dies.

In the section in which I outlined some of the causes of asthma I described some of the things that can make wheezing worse. It is obviously wise, therefore, to try and ensure that these irritants are avoided whenever possible. Cigarette smoking is probably the worst irritant of all and few things parents can do to help their children's asthma will prove more effective than giving up smoking!

There are no drugs or medicines that can be bought over the counter that I recommend for the asthmatic child. You really are wasting your money if you try buying any magic remedies that you see advertised.

There are, however, some very effective drugs available on prescription. Some of these are intended to help relieve the symptoms of asthma while others are intended to help prevent the symptoms developing. Drugs that fall into the first category must usually be given only when symptoms are present while drugs which fall into the second category must obviously be given regularly if they're to work at all. It is, therefore, vital that parents of asthmatic children know as much as possible about their children's disorders. And when drugs are prescribed it is sensible to make sure that you know whether the drugs are curative or prophylactic.

It is also important to make sure that you keep a good supply of medicine in stock so that you don't run out unexpectedly. Attacks of asthma often seem to start at night, at weekends or when you are on holiday. You'll save a lot of time and energy (and a good deal of worry) if you keep a small emergency stock of whatever drugs your child needs. Keep an eye on the 'expiry date' on the label.

Finally, I must point out that although the temptation is to wrap a child with asthma in cotton wool there is nothing worse. Overprotected children tend to suffer more because they start worrying themselves. There is no reason why an asthmatic child shouldn't lead a perfectly normal, active life whenever the wheezing is under control. And for the majority of children that will be most of the time.

When should we see the doctor?
Any child who is breathless or who wheezes either regularly or persistently needs to be examined by a doctor. Even if you recognise that your child has asthma and you know exactly what to do for him it's probably a good idea just to visit your doctor. That will at least ensure that if you need emergency help he'll know something about the child's medical history.

Bad breath

What is it?

Bad breath (or halitosis) doesn't really need much in the way of introduction. I don't think it needs to be regarded as a medical problem unless it is persistent or recurrent. Bad breath is persistent if it lasts for more than one day or if it remains noticeable after the most probable, common causes have been eliminated.

What causes it?

Catarrh, sinusitis, infected gums, dirty teeth, indigestion and constipation are just some of the common causes of bad breath.

How do we make the diagnosis?

Easily.

What can we do about it?

The treatment depends upon the cause. If you think your child has any of the problems listed above then consult the appropriate page for suitable advice. Good dental care is probably the simplest and most effective way to deal with the majority of cases of bad breath (see page 283). Mouthwashes sold commercially usually contain a mixture of antiseptics while breath fresheners usually consist of a mixture of alcohol, water and artificial sweeteners. You can make your own mouthwash quite simply by putting half a teaspoonful of salt into a glass of warm water. To make the mouthwash a little more palatable you can try adding a drop of peppermint oil to the glass of water.

When do we need to see the doctor?

If a child's bad breath does not improve when you have dealt with all the underlying problems which you think could be involved you should seek medical advice. You should also seek medical advice if the bad breath is accompanied by any other symptoms.

Baldness (alopecia)

What is it?
A complete or partial absence of hair on the head. Some children are born bald and stay bald, others are born with a head full of hair and then become bald.

What causes it?
Very, very rarely a child may be born bald and stay bald. This type of congenital baldness is, however, extremely uncommon. The same is true of congenital baldness in which a baby is born with a full head of hair but gradually loses its hair never to have it replaced.

One of the commonest causes of baldness in children is a condition called alopecia areata. This is a quite startling disorder since the hair literally does fall out in handfuls leaving great round or oval patches of scalp entirely bare. The bald bare scalp looks slightly pink and fresh. This condition usually affects only patches of the scalp but very occasionally it may affect the whole head. The eyebrows and eyelashes are also sometimes affected. There is no known cause for this condition but it is widely believed that it is a consequence of stress and anxiety. And just as there is no known cause so there is no known cure. What we do know is that the condition usually clears itself up remarkably successfully. Most of the people who have suffered from alopecia areata have a full head of hair again within a matter of months if not weeks.

The other common cause of baldness in children is ringworm. Again this produces scattered bald spots. With ringworm, however, the bald spots are rather scaly and the patches are littered with the broken-off ends of hair.

There are some temporary problems which exist and I think I should perhaps mention them briefly. First of all there are all number of babies who will lose some of their hair by rubbing their heads on the bottom of their playpen or cot. That hair loss is very temporary. Then there are those children who favour very tight hairstyles such as old fashioned pigtails, pony tails, braids and so on. These styles involve pulling the hair back tightly from the front of the head and as a result a condition known as 'traction alopecia' can result. This isn't anything to worry about but it is probably wise to change the hairstyle at least temporarily. And finally in this group I must mention the fact that some children have a habit of playing with their hair and twisting it between their fingers while others have a strange habit of literally pulling out hair in handfuls. Obviously, in both these cases the hair will grow again if given the opportunity.

The only other type of hair loss which is really likely to affect children is the gradual, natural loss of hair which continues all the time on a normal scalp. Older children sometimes notice that their combs and hair brushes are suddenly being filled with hair and so they become convinced that they are going bald. This is an entirely normal phenomenon and is merely a manifestation of the variations which exist in normal people.

What can we do about it?
Unless the baldness is caused by a hairstyle or by some habit that can be broken there isn't much that you can do at home about bald patches. Don't waste money on over-the-counter preparations or on visiting beauty specialists of any kind.

When do we need to see the doctor?
You should visit the doctor if you notice bald patches developing. It is important to differentiate between alopecia areata and ringworm since although the former condition doesn't require any treatment the latter does.

Bedwetting

What is it?
Enuresis is officially defined as the frequent passage of urine in inappropriate circumstances by a child who has no responsible organic disease. Before being described as enuretic a child must have either reached an age at which bladder control is usually developed or have achieved control of his bladder for a while and lost it again.

The type of enuresis which causes most problems and most heartache is bedwetting; a condition in which the child wets his or her bed at night either on a regular basis or at least often enough for the events to be regarded as seriously disturbing the size of the household wash.

Are boys or girls usually affected?
Bedwetting can affect both boys and girls but it is commoner in boys.

Is it hereditary?
Yes, there does seem to be a hereditary link. Children whose parents wet the bed at an age when they should have been dry are more likely to suffer from bedwetting.

How is control usually obtained?
The infant's bladder has an inbuilt reflex which is designed to automatically empty the contents whenever the bladder is fully distended with urine. Although this reflex has a vital function there are obvious social disadvantages to such a system and so we are all encouraged to try and obtain some sort of control over our bladders.

Young children rarely get control over their bladders before they can walk. By the age of about eighteen months, however, most are beginning to indicate that they are about to pass urine. Gradually, over the months which follow, they get more skilled at recognising that they need to pass urine. If these early signs are recognised and encouraged by the parents then the child will soon learn to become aware of the sensation that the bladder (or indeed the bowel) needs emptying.

Daytime control comes first. Nighttime control will usually come a little later.

At what age is night time control usually obtained?
Three quarters of all children are dry at night by the age of $3^1/_2$ years. Nine out of ten children are dry at night by the time they reach the age of 5 years.

What causes bedwetting?
Occasional bedwetting is by no means exceptional. All children will occasionally lose control of their bladders during the night and even during the day when they are excited, ill or tired. Many adults (particularly women) will confirm that this is a problem which is by no means confined to children.

But when the problem becomes regular then bedwetting needs to be taken seriously.

One of the commonest causes is anxiety, stress, distress, worry or fear. Bedwetting is fairly common among young children who are starting school for the first time, for example. When that happens and the bedwetting doesn't last for more than a month or so then nothing needs to be done about it.

When bedwetting persists and there are no obvious psychological problems it is sometimes worth looking at the facilities which exist at night-time. Many children are frightened to go to the toilet by themselves in the dark, particularly if the lavatory is a long way from their bedroom, if they cannot reach the light switch, or if they are frightened of falling into the lavatory pan. It may be a good idea to put a small potty into the child's bedroom and to provide a night light or table lamp.

Sometimes a child will be wet at night because his parents have put so much pressure on him and have so emphasised the importance of night-time dryness that he is terrified of failing. That terror produces stress which produces bedwetting.

In a fairly small number of cases there will be a genuine physical cause. The child with an infection in his bladder or kidneys will only gain control when the infection has been cleared up. And the diabetic child will only gain control when his diabetes has been controlled.

In the majority of cases, however, there is no simple specific answer. It may be that the child's bladder is unusually small and sensitive and that his urine output is unusually large. Whatever the cause it is important to remember that most children will eventually gain total control of their bladders.

When should we see the doctor?
You should seek medical advice if:
1 Your child is over 5 years old and wet at night.
2 Your child is over the age of 2 and is still wet all the time – both day and night – and there doesn't seem to be any sign of him gaining control.
3 Your child did have good bladder control both during the daytime and at night and now seems to have lost that control.

What can we do about it?
You don't need to do anything about it if your child only wets the bed occasionally. If, however, the bedwetting is a fairly frequent problem but your child has good control in the daytime there are several things you can try before visiting the doctor.

There are many conflicting pieces of advice in the medical textbooks and many paediatricians will argue about the best methods to deal with bedwetting. I've tried to find a consensus of opinion and to look for the logical, sensible ideas.

I suggest that you should try lifting your child out of bed at about 10 p.m. and taking him along to the toilet and I also suggest that you resist the temptation to limit fluids in the evenings. The consensus of opinion seems to be that this just doesn't work and it just makes the child feel that he is being punished.

It is probably a good idea to try and persuade your child to hold his urine for as long as possible during the daytime since that will probably help expand the bladder and improve control and it is also undoubtedly a good idea to prepare a chart or calendar on which your child can mark off his dry nights and wet nights. Use coloured stickers to illustrate the dry nights and leave the child's pride to do the rest. Encouragement and support will help much more than punishment.

On a purely practical level it is probably wise to leave your child in nappies until he is consistently dry at night and to use rubber sheets and absorbent mats to help limit the amount of extra laundry. If the lavatory is a long way from the child's bedroom then put a potty inside the room and make sure that there is a light within reach of the bed.

What will the doctor do?
If you take your child to a doctor and explain that he has not got good bladder control then the doctor will usually begin by testing the child's urine. This will hopefully show up any sign of diabetes or any sign of infection. The doctor will probably also want to check for any signs of any physical abnormality.

Assuming that he doesn't find any physical or psychological problems which he considers responsible the doctor may then decide either to treat your child himself or may decide to refer him to a specialist. There are some specialist clinics at which teams of doctors and nurses do nothing else but deal with children who have had difficulty in acquiring bladder control.

There are two types of medical treatment usually offered. One of the most popular techniques is to use an enuresis alarm. This consist of a special pad which is put under the child's sheet at night. When urine leaks out and wets the pad the circuit is broken and a buzzer sounds. The buzzer switch should be far

enough from the bed to ensure that the child has to get out of bed
to turn off the alarm. Hopefully he will empty his bladder in some
more appropriate place while he is up out of bed switching off
the alarm.

Those who have had most success with these alarms suggest
that they should be used for several weeks before being
discarded (as either successful or useless). They suggest that a
child should have been dry for three to four weeks before the
alarm is disconnected and the mat removed. It is very important
to make sure that the buzzer can't be switched off without the
child getting up out of bed.

The other treatment doctors sometimes offer involves drugs.
There are various different products available and there is much
medical controversy over the safety and efficacy of these
substances. However safe and effective these products are they
certainly shouldn't be used unless they are a last resort.

Birthmarks

What are they?

There are many different types of birthmark. The only thing that
these skin lesions have in common is that they are all visible!
(They are not even all present at birth as the name might suggest
for the type of mark known as a cavernous haemangioma
sometimes only becomes apparent a week or two after the baby's
birth.)

What causes them?

Birthmarks are the result of slight flaws in the development
process. Some marks result from flaws in the development of
blood vessels while others are the result of flaws in the
distribution of skin pigments.

How can we tell what sort of birthmark our child has?

It is always worthwhile showing a mark to your doctor and asking
for his advice and comments. You don't need to make a special
journey to the surgery to do this unless the mark has changed in
any way or has started to bleed. Just show the doctor when you
visit for some other reason.

You should, however, be able to identify some of the

commonest types of birthmark yourself without too much difficulty. The type of mark known as the cavernous haemangioma is perhaps more widely known as a strawberry birthmark. This name is genuinely useful in that it offers a good basic description of the mark. The lesion is usually pink or bright red and it is clearly raised above the level of the skin so that it almost looks like a strawberry struggling to escape. Strawberry birthmarks can appear anywhere on the body and for the first few months of a child's life they continue to grow steadily in size. They look very dramatic and can be most worrying for parents who have never seen anything like them before. By the time a child reaches the age of 10, however, most of these birthmarks will have disappeared completely. There is not usually any need for either surgical or medical treatment. About ten per cent of all babies seem to have strawberry birthmarks.

Another common lesion that usually disappears by itself is the blue-grey discolouration which is sometimes visible and which looks rather like a bruise. Known as Mongolian spots, these lesions are commonest at the base of the spine. They are found most frequently on babies with darker skins. These marks have nothing to do with mongolism and they usually disappear by the time the child reaches the age of 4.

The marks known as naevus simplex (and also sometimes called salmon patches, angels kisses or stork bites) are light red areas which also tend to disappear spontaneously – usually within twelve months or so.

The commonest type of birthmarks that don't disappear themselves are the capillary haemangiomas. Known as port wine stains because they are flat, purple and do indeed look as though they have been made by the spilling of some rich, red liquid they occur most commonly on the face – usually affecting one side only.

What can we do?

There is obviously no need to do anything at all about birthmarks which fade by themselves but birthmarks which don't fade – such as port wine stains – can be quite worrying. The only really effective remedy is to use waterproof cosmetic camouflage creams. A specialist beautician or dermatologist will usually be able to explain how best to mix different colours so as to produce a cream which most effectively matches the patient's own skin.

When do we need to see a doctor?

You should always ask a doctor for routine advice about any birthmark. But you should seek advice without delay if any birthmark changes shape, size or colour, bleeds or changes in any other way.

Bites and stings

What causes them?

Bees, wasps, jellyfish and nettles sting. Animals, snakes, mosquitoes, gnats, fleas, lice and ticks bite.

What can we do about them?

1 Bee stings The unique fact about bee stings is that when the bee has sunk its stinger into the skin it cannot withdraw it again. It disembowels itself leaving behind the barb and the venom sac. The sac continues to discharge venom into the victim long after the bee has flown away and the stinger is actually driven further into the skin. Since drop for drop the venom of the bee is said to be just as potent as that of the rattlesnake it is obviously important to try and get the sac out of the skin as soon as possible.

It's best not to try and do this by pulling the barb straight out of the skin with your finger nails since there is a good chance that you'll only squeeze the remaining venom into the skin. It is much safer to try and tease the stinger out sideways, using a sterilised needle or a pair of eyebrow tweezers. If you can't see what you're doing then use a magnifying glass to enlarge the area you're looking at.

Once the stinger and venom sac have been removed there isn't a lot more that you can do. A cold dressing, a dash of calamine lotion or a piece of ice will do as much good as anything else. If the sting is in the mouth you can give a sodium bicarbonate mouthwash.

2 Wasp stings Unlike the bee the wasp retains its barb after an attack and can sting again. This has disadvantages for other potential victims but means that the person who has been stung will not receive any more venom from that particular sting.

There is no specific treatment for a single wasp sting but a cold dressing, a dash of calamine lotion or a piece of ice will probably do as much good as anything else. I don't recommend antihistamine creams because they can produce allergic reactions of their own.

3 Jellyfish stings If the sting has only a minor localised effect there is no need to do anything other than apply the usual cold dressing or dash of calamine lotion. You should cover your hands with some sort of protection when picking off any pieces of jellyfish which are still sticking to your child. The Portuguese Man of War is the most dangerous jellyfish and if you think your child has been stung by one of those you should seek medical advice. Warning signs and notices are usually put up when bathing waters are infested with jellyfish and these should obviously be regarded seriously.

4 Nettle stings Nettle stings are uncomfortable but rarely serious. If you can't get hold of calamine lotion or a cold dressing you can try the old remedy of rubbing the stinging area with a dock leaf. This will often relieve the irritation very effectively.

5 Animal bites The child who has been bitten by an animal will usually be very upset and distraught. Your first task therefore is to calm him as much as you possibly can. You should also protect the child from any further bites. Since animal bites can introduce infection into the skin it's important to clean the wound as soon as possible either with plenty of running water or with a liquid antiseptic. Because of the risk of contracting tetanus it is important for any unprotected child to have a vaccination jab (see page 308). Animal bites are rarely large or serious but because of the risk of infection it is usually wise to obtain medical advice.

6 Snake bites If the snake which has done the biting is a non-poisonous variety then the bite should be treated in the same way as an animal bite. If, however, the snake is poisonous, or could be poisonous, then the best solution is to seek medical attention immediately. You should try to keep the child calm and quiet and you should, if possible, cool the bitten area with ice or cold water. Some experts claim that if the snake is poisonous you should tie a tourniquet above the bite, make two incisions over the site of the bite and suck out the poison. Others claim that this dramatic form of treatment is not only unnecessary but also dangerous. I suspect that unless you're a long way from a medical centre and a well-trained first-aid expert it is probably better to settle for obtaining medical help as soon as possible.

Incidentally it is a good idea to try and catch and kill the snake so that it can be identified.

7 Mosquitoes and gnats The cold dressing and calamine lotion are the best forms of treatment for bites by these insects. It is wise to try and stop the child from scratching the bitten areas since any scratching will increase the risk of infection. If the mosquito bites were contracted in any area where malaria is known then you should seek medical advice as soon as possible. You should also seek medical advice if any unexpected symptoms or complications arise within the subsequent six months.

8 Fleas, lice, ticks, bedbugs There is no specific treatment for bites made by any of these small creatures. All you can do is use calamine and cold dressings to soothe the inflamed area. You will, of course, want to get rid of the responsible creatures.

Fleas, in particular, can be very difficult to eradicate. Even when they are caught they can be difficult to kill. Holding them under water and drowning them or flushing them away sound extreme but is often the only effective method of extermination.

If you have a family pet then that should be examined by a vet since fleas in particular can move from animals to humans.

When should we see the doctor?
Obviously when individual bites and stings seem particularly large or uncomfortable medical advice should be sought without delay. And, as I have already suggested, it is always wise to seek medical advice for animal or snake bites.

It is, in addition, important to be aware that children can sometimes have allergic reactions to otherwise insignificant bites and stings.

In just the same way that some individuals can be allergic to strawberries or penicillin so others can have allergic reactions to wasp or bee stings. In these cases the reaction is much more generalised than the localised reddening, burning and itching of the skin that we usually associate with a bee or wasp sting. The patient may well be short of breath, restless, blue and even unconscious. He will almost certainly have a generalised skin rash and be both weak and nauseous.

Allergy reactions can develop very quickly and the sting victim can change from being quite healthy to looking very ill indeed within the space of a few minutes. It is usually very obvious that medical attention is needed.

If you think that a child of yours is having an allergy reaction to an insect sting or bite then you should either take him straight to the local casualty department or straight to your local doctor. If you have no transport available then telephone the emergency services and your own doctor for immediate help. The doctor will inject either an antihistamine or a type of adrenalin and in the majority of cases the recovery will be swift and dramatic.

It is also important to seek medical advice straight away if a child has been bitten near to the mouth, or in any other place where a swelling seems to be growing to dangerous proportions, or if the child has been bitten a number of times. A child who has received many injections of wasp or bee venom may have received so much poison that he may be at risk.

What can we do to protect our child?

Generally speaking it is, of course, quite impossible to protect your child against all risks of being bitten or stung. And the consequences of an isolated bite or sting are rarely serious enough to warrant any restrictions which you might consider.

When, however, a child has been shown to have developed an allergy to bee or wasp venom then it is extremely important to take precautions. Any additional future exposure to venom could prove fatal.

Apart from the fact that it is obviously wise to do all that you can to protect your child from bees and wasps if he is allergic to them it is also sensible to ask your doctor to provide you with a supply of antihistamine tablets and, possibly, with an ampoule containing either adrenalin or an antihistamine and a syringe and needle.

Recently new vaccines have come on to the market which can be used to protect susceptible children against bee and wasp stings. These are only recommended for use on individuals whose previous reactions have been severe but there seems a very good chance that the protection they provide will be extremely useful.

Bleeding

What is it?

Blood is pumped around the body in a continuous circle. It is
pumped into the lungs where it picks up fresh supplies of oxygen
and to the intestinal tract where it picks up the substances the
body has extracted from food supplies. It is then pumped around
the rest of the body so that the oxygen and food can be
distributed to the tissues. A special sequence of vessels takes
blood along to the kidneys so that waste material can be
removed prior to excretion in the urine.

The vessels which carry freshly oxygenated blood to the
tissues have thicker walls than any others. These are the arteries
and the blood they carry is under a considerable amount of
pressure. The vessels through which blood returns from the
tissues to the heart and lungs are the veins. Here the blood is
under much less pressure and it travels far less quickly. The
veins are, consequently, thinner-walled and weaker than the
arteries.

The smallest vessels of all are the capillaries which make up
the enormous network of tiny vessels connecting together the
arteries and the veins. It is through the thin and fragile walls of
the capillaries that oxygen and foodstuffs filter out into the tissues
and waste products filter back into the blood supply.

Of these three types of vessel the capillaries are the weakest
and easiest to damage while the arteries are the strongest and
most difficult to damage. The effect of any damage obviously
varies too and whereas damage to a few small capillaries may
produce nothing more than a small bruise, damage to a large
artery will result in blood being lost in great quantities and at
tremendous rate. Arterial damage is relatively rare and may be
extremely serious. The frequency and seriousness of vein
damage falls somewhere between those two extremes.

The blood supply is, of course, extremely vital to the human
organism. And although fresh supplies of all blood cells can be
produced, and are produced continually to replace those which
are lost through natural wastage, the body has a number of
complex mechanisms which are designed solely to ensure that
after any injury blood loss is minimised.

The clotting mechanisms which ensure that at the site of any wound blood loss is kept to a minimum and any tissue damage or vessel damage is repaired with a blood clot are designed to come into operation after a short delay. This helps ensure that the wound site is washed clear by the initial flow of blood.

Under normal circumstances, therefore, the human body is perfectly well equipped to deal with a minor injury which threatens to cause a minor loss of blood. There are, however, circumstances which may lower the efficiency of the blood clotting mechanism.

To begin with if the wound size is too great the body's clotting mechanism will be of little use. A clot can form over a fairly small area and can restrict blood loss very effectively. But if the area is a large one the clot will be swept aside as fast as it is made. The same sort of thing happens if the vessel that has been in jured is a large artery. When this is the case the rate and force of blood loss may be so great that the clotting mechanism will just not be able to cope.

You may be able to stop a leaky pipe with a piece of gum but if the water pressure is too high or the size of the hole too large the gum will quickly get washed to one side.

There are also some disorders which specifically affect the clotting mechanism. In haemophilia, for example, not all the ingredients for clot making are present in the blood. When the clot making mechanism is disrupted even a comparatively mild injury can prove fatal. A small cut that would be quickly stopped by a clot in a normal, healthy individual may result in a steady, continual loss of blood for days or even weeks.

What's the difference between internal and external bleeding?
Obviously the blood vessels which supply the skin and outer tissues of the body are much more easily damaged than the vessels which are buried deep inside the body. It is also easier to see when the outer vessels are damaged and much easier to do something to prevent the loss of blood.

Internal bleeding can occur with or without there having been any external signs of damage. If, for example, an individual is hit on the head it is possible for there to be severe internal bleeding and little or no external sign of any damage. Similarly a blow to the abdomen may leave no sign at all of any external damage but may cause serious internal bleeding.

How do we tell when there is serious internal bleeding?
If after an injury or accident your child becomes pale, sweaty, sleepy or breathless then you should consider the possibility of internal bleeding and request medical advice immediately.

How can we help stop bleeding?
In an emergency when blood is being lost at a great rate the most effective form of first aid is the simplest. All you have to do is to press as hard as you can on the bleeding point. If you have time to make a nice neat pad out of some piece of freshly laundered material that is fine but if you don't have time to find a pad on which to press it doesn't matter: just press directly on to the wound. The risks of any infection developing as a result of your intervention are far smaller than the risks the patient runs from blood loss.

To slow down bleeding in one particular part of the body it helps to raise that part of the body as far above the rest of the body as possible. This works by simple gravity! So, for example, if you have a patient with a wound in the hand you will be able to slow down blood loss considerably by raising the child's hand as high as possible above his head. If the wound is on the foot lie the patient down and raise his foot in the air.

Once any clots have formed don't be tempted to pick them off because they look unsightly. They are there for a purpose and should be left undisturbed as long as possible.

When should we see a doctor?
You must obviously seek medical advice if a wound looks as though it will need stitching or closing by a doctor in any other way. You may be able to seal wounds under one inch in length at home with sticking plasters but anything longer than that will almost certainly require suturing.

You should seek medical advice straight away if your child becomes pale, sweaty, sleepy or breathless. Those symptoms suggest that blood loss is becoming serious.

You should also see a doctor if for any reason bleeding doesn't stop within ten or fifteen minutes.

You should obviously see a doctor if there is any family history of a bleeding disorder. Most bleeding disorders are inherited and so there will usually be some such history.

If a wound looks dirty or was obtained out of doors you should

seek medical advice so that a tetanus injection can be given.
Details of vaccination programmes against tetanus are given on
page 308.

What will the doctor do?
The action your doctor takes will obviously depend upon the site
and extent of the bleeding. If the blood loss has been dramatic
the doctors may arrange for a blood transfusion or may boost the
circulation with simple fluids. If the bleeding vessel is easy to see
and repair, simple suturing or cautery may be all that is required.
If, however, the bleeding is internal then an operation may be
needed.

Examining the blood pressure, taking the pulse and looking at
the blood in a laboratory will all help the doctor decide on the
appropriate form of treatment.

If a child has one of the inherited bleeding disorders he may
need special treatment. If that is the case you will normally be
provided with the telephone number and address of one of the
special centres where doctors specialise in the treatment of your
child's condition.

Blindness

What types of blindness are there?
Total blindness is relatively rare among children but there are
very many children with extremely poor vision. These children
are officially classified as partially sighted but in practical terms
they often share the same short of general handicaps as children
who are completely blind.

How do we make the diagnosis?
If a baby's eyes continually move from side to side without ever
settling in one place then there may be something wrong.
Similarly if older babies cannot follow objects with their eyes
there may be a visual difficulty. Usually babies have jerky eye
movements but can follow a stimulus reasonably well. Horizontal
eye movements are usually better in the first few months of life
than vertical eye movements.

Up to the age of two months it is of course extremely difficult to
test a baby's eyes but even at that early stage most babies will

turn towards the light and will follow a human face at a distance of about two feet. Between two months and six months of age babies can usually recognise their parents and some special objects. Over the age of six months infants should be able to start picking up objects and should have normal eye movements.

In the section on page 220 I have described another common and worrying problem – the squint.

What causes blindness?

Cataracts are among the commoner causes of complete or nearly complete blindness. These can be inherited and they can be caused if the child's mother contracts certain infections (such as german measles) during her pregnancy. Some children have a type of glaucoma causing blindness while others may suffer from any one of a number of rare disorders such as a tumour.

In children who were not born blind but who have become blind injury and infection are two of the commoner causes. Of the infections which cause a loss of vision toxocara is one of the most important. This worm infestation can be caught from dogs and cats and picked up by playing on fouled grass (see page 254).

Whatever the cause of a child's blindness may be it is important to make the diagnosis as soon as possible so that any suitable treatment can be started without delay and so that the child can benefit from the special types of attention and training which are available.

What about colour blindness?

This is something of a misnomer because the colour-blind child isn't blind in any true sense of the word. He will, however, have difficulty in distinguishing between certain colours which to the normal eye appear quite different. It is usually reds and greens which get mixed up. Colour blindness is an inherited disorder and it is commoner among boys than girls. Usually it is mild and only of real significance if the child tries to follow a career where it is important that he be able to distinguish accurately between all colours. Flying is one career that usually seems an impractical choice for the colour-blind child.

What is astigmatism?

In this condition the cornea is slightly misshapen and the result is that when the eye is focused on one particular line other lines which are at right angles to it will appear blurred. The condition can usually be corrected with the aid of suitable spectacles.

What can we do to help our blind child?

1 You must get in touch with the experts. There are many specialists who spend their lives working with the blind and the partially sighted and whose experience and equipment can be used to great advantage. Your own family doctor will be the best person to put you in touch with these experts.

2 Blind children need to have their other senses stimulated more than other children if they are to develop properly. In practice the opposite often happens and blind children are frequently protected from the world by worried parents. Overprotection invariably leads to deprivation of normal sensory material. Blind children should be taught and encouraged to do things for themselves. It is difficult to hold back and not help a blind child do up buttons, brush his teeth and so on but only by doing just this, and allowing the blind child to learn how to do things for himself, will he gain true independence.

The blind child needs to use his ears, his mouth and his fingers in place of his eyes and so he should be allowed to touch and feel things wherever this is possible.

3 To help a blind child learn the names of objects it is essential to say the names when he is handling them so that he learns to associate the name with the feel of the object.

4 When a blind child reaches the age at which he might be expected to be learning how to read he should be taught braille. It is also a good idea to teach him how to touch type since this will enable him to communicate by letter with people who can see. Modern electrical equipment is often of tremendous value, with tape and cassette recorders being particularly valuable.

5 It is vital to remember that a blind or partially sighted child needs the same amount of discipline and the same firm handling as any other child. He needs understanding but it is important not to allow sympathy and pity to intrude on the relationship.

6 All babies and young children like routine and fixed habits. Blind babies and young children respond particularly well to routine. This provides them with a considerable amount of vital security.

7 Feeding is sometimes difficult for blind children. The problems are obvious enough if you think about them. If, for example, a

child puts down a biscuit he is eating he may not be able to find it
again.

8 Since blind children cannot comment on what they see around
them they tend to be slow to speak. They need plenty of
encouragement and parents should talk to them as often as
possible, preferably describing what they are doing and what the
child is touching. Story telling is obviously important and to the
developing blind child records and tapes serve the same function
as the story book for the sighted child.

9 Blind children are often very frightened by sudden noises or
by noises which they don't understand. Try and explain where
you can and try and warn your child if, for example, you are
about to switch on the washing machine or vacuum cleaner.

10 Blind children are usually of normal intelligence. There is no
reason at all to assume that because a child cannot see properly
his brain is in any way adversely affected. Do remember this
when you are talking to him and try to avoid being patronising or
condescending.

11 If you are leaving a room in which a blind child is settled then
do warn him. Otherwise he may suddenly say something
expecting you to be there. This can be very frightening.

Boils

What are they?

The body is covered with thousands of very tiny hairs. Each of
these tiny hairs grows through the skin from a follicle. If one of
these follicles becomes infected then a swollen, painful, hot,
localised, red lump can develop. That is a boil.

Similarly if a sweat gland, a sebaceous gland or even a small
cut in the skin becomes infected the result may be a boil. A
pimple or spot, by the way, is just an underdeveloped boil.

Boils most commonly develop where the skin is rubbed by the
clothing and that is why they seem to develop most frequently in
places that are most troublesome! The back of the neck where
the collar rubs is a common site for boils.

What can we do about them?

The first thing is to stop your child squeezing the boil. This is just
as likely to send the pus downwards and into the tissues

surrounding the boil as to send the pus upwards and out into the open.

The best treatment is the simplest. Just cover the boil with a dry dressing and then leave it alone to come to a head and burst. Traditionally it is thought that boils need to be covered with special pastes in order to draw them. My feeling is that the only useful and necessary treatment is warmth. Put a wrapped hot-water bottle over the dressed boil and not only will the boil be encouraged to burst but the pain will be relieved.

Once the boil has burst all you need to do is change the dressing, being careful to burn each old dressing as quickly as possible and to wash the skin surrounding the boil.

Are they infectious?
Yes. Boils are made up of bacteria and live and dead cells. The matter from a boil is extremely infectious. To make sure that the patient does not develop additional boils it is important to clean the area around a boil carefully with soap and water or with a liquid antiseptic.

There is no point in using any special cream or ointment.

What is a carbuncle?
A carbuncle is simply a large boil with a number of heads. Alternatively it can be described as a number of boils situated very close together.

What is a stye?
A boil on the edge of the eyelid.

What is an abscess?
A boil is usually confined to the skin. A collection of pus in other tissues or organs (such as muscle or bone) is called an abscess. Because they are often denied direct access to the outside world abscesses are sometimes more difficult to drain than boils.

How can we prevent boils developing?
If your child suffers from recurrent boils then one member of the family is probably acting as a carrier. A nose swab from each member of the family is usually a good idea since the organisms responsible often live in the nostrils.

Any child who suffers from boils should have his or her urine tested for sugar since diabetes is a condition which makes the development of boils more likely.

When do we need to see the doctor?
If a boil or carbuncle becomes very large and very painful and doesn't look like bursting by itself your doctor may be able to incise and drain it. When he has done that he may take a sample from the boil in order to identify the responsible organism.

If the boil is in a very difficult and painful position or is on or around the eye and seems to be growing to a size you consider dangerous then you should also seek medical advice.

You should see a doctor if red lines appear on the skin around a boil since these may suggest that the infection is spreading.

Most doctors don't prescribe antibiotics for most boils since these infections will usually clear up by themselves. Antibiotics can, indeed, make things worse by sealing off the boil.

Bow legs

What are they?
The legs are bowed so that the knees seem to be a long way apart.

What causes it?
This is an entirely normal condition in babies and young children. Although overweight children may seem to have bowed legs for slightly longer than others, it is normal for bowed legs to straighten by the time a child reaches the age of 5 unless there is some underlying disorder of the bones.

Rickets is the disease most commonly associated with a bowing of the legs. This is a relatively rare condition in the developed countries of the world. It is caused by a deficiency of vitamin D. There are also some relatively rare orthopaedic problems which can cause bowing.

When do we need to see the doctor?
1 If there seems to be bowing of one leg but not of the other then you should seek medical advice.
2 If when your child can stand there is more than half an inch separating the knees when the ankles are touching.

3 If your child's shoes seem to be wearing out unevenly or you have noticed any significant difficulty in walking.

What will he do?
He will arrange for tests and X-rays designed to show whether or not there is any serious cause for the bowing. If there is then an orthopaedic surgeon may be asked to provide a brace or consider surgical help.

Breast problems

What are they?
The only time boys are likely to be worried by their breasts is when they become clearly visible! This condition – known as gynaecomastia – is fairly common among boys at puberty and it isn't usually anything to worry about. If everything else is developing normally then the breast enlargement will usually disappear after a few admittedly embarrassing months. Some- times boys who are overweight will appear to have well- developed breasts because of the folds of fat on their chests. These boys may need to lose weight before they regain a more masculine shape.

Girls, of course, are exposed to a far wider range of problems.

1 Their breasts are too small Girls reach puberty at different ages and while one girl in a class may have fully developed adult shape breasts other girls may have hardly anything to put into a bra. Usually a girl whose breasts have not properly developed will also be lagging behind in other areas too – she is unlikely to have started her periods, for example. Reassurance may need to be offered regularly.

Sometimes, of course, even when a girl has finished growing and has acquired all the other signs of early womanhood she'll still consider that her breasts are too small. However irrational these fears may be they should not be ridiculed. Growing girls are extremely sensitive about their figures and if reassurance doesn't satisfy them then they should be offered practical professional advice.

2 Their breasts are too large Girls whose breasts develop

quicker than those of their peers at school will often suffer just as much embarrassment as girls with no breast development. This embarrassment is, however, usually short-lived. Much more long-lasting is the type of anxiety girls suffer when their breasts overdevelop. Any girl whose breasts are so large that they produce backache, chafing and other problems should receive genuine advice. The psychological problems associated with mammary hypertrophy (over-large breasts) usually far exceed the physical problems.

3 Their breasts are lumpy There are all sorts of innocent explanations for lumps in the breast. Serious problems are extremely rare among young girls. Nevertheless no lump, however slight or apparently insignificant, should be left. You should teach your daughter to seek professional advice whenever she feels or finds a lump or swelling of any kind.

4 Their breasts are unequal in size Breasts, like all paired organs, tend to be of different sizes. Very few women have breasts which are identical. If the difference is very noticeable (or the girl feels that the difference is very noticeable) then she should be seen by her family doctor and preferably by a plastic surgeon too.

5 They have extra nipples This is a problem which may affect boys as well as girls. It is nothing to worry about. The accessory nipples can easily be removed by a surgeon.

Breath holding

What is it?
Children between the ages of 1 and 5 will sometimes deliberately hold their breath until they become limp, blue and even unconscious.

What causes it?
Breath holding attacks are not caused by any abnormality and they do not cause any physical damage. They simply result from the child's deliberate refusal to breathe! Although breath holding attacks sometimes follow pain or fear they are usually the result of the child being hurt, frustrated, thwarted or annoyed. Breath

holding attacks are in fact nothing more than very frightening,
very effective temper tantrums.

Are breath holding attacks dangerous?
Breath holding attacks are frightening but they aren't really
dangerous. If the child holds his breath long enough he will
eventually go unconscious and start breathing again automatically. The main risk is that the lack of oxygen to the brain can
produce a convulsion.

What can we do about it?
There isn't a lot you can do to abort an attack that is already
taking place. There certainly does not seem to be a lot of point in
threatening or slapping a child who is breath holding. If the
attack has only just started you may be able to prevent it
developing by hooking your finger over his tongue and pulling
the tongue forwards. Alternatively you can try splashing a little
cold water in his face.

The most important thing to remember is that you must not give
in to the child who holds his breath in an attempt to force you to
do something or to let him do something. You should try and
keep calm and you should try and ignore the attack as much as
you can. The parent whose child discovers that breath holding is
a good way to exert influence will find that the ploy is used more
and more often.

Most children quickly learn that breath holding doesn't pay and
stop it.

When do we need to see the doctor?
It is not always easy to distinguish between breath holding
attacks and fits. If you are at all uncertain then seek medical
advice.

Breathlessness

What causes it?
Some causes of breathlessness are mild, insignificant and self-
limiting. Others are serious and require a good deal of
specialised attention.

Into the first category of disorders fall those minor childhood ailments such as the common cold, catarrh, sinus problems and simple chest infections. Into the second category fall those more worrying ailments which involve major organs such as the lungs and heart.

How do we make the diagnosis?
If you are certain that your child's breathlessness is caused by a minor problem then there is no need to seek medical advice. If you suspect that the problem may be more serious, if you are not certain that the problem is a minor one or if the child is in distress then you should seek medical advice without delay.

What can we do about it?
Whatever the cause may be, breathlessness is an extremely frightening symptom for both the patient and for any observers. Since anxiety and fear make almost all types of breathlessness worse it is important for parents to reassure and comfort their breathless child. Staying calm may be difficult but it is the most important thing that a parent can do.

If breathing stops altogether then artificial respiration should be tried. Details are on page 5. If breathlessness accompanies other minor symptoms (such as wheezing, cough, stuffiness and so on) then treatment should be designed to cope with those symptoms too.

When should we see the doctor?
You should see the doctor if your child's breathlessness is caused by anything other than a minor respiratory infection or if the amount of breathlessness causes anxiety or distress.

What will the doctor do?
The investigations and type of treatment offered will obviously vary very much according to the cause of the breathlessness.

Broken bones (fractures)

How do we make the diagnosis?
If a bone is broken there will obviously be pain and a good deal of tenderness. Some deformity of the bone will probably be visible; if it isn't visible then you should be able to feel the

deformity. The child will not be able to use the broken bone properly and there will also usually be swelling at the side of the break.

Distinguishing between a broken bone and a sprain is not always easy but whereas the child with a sprain will usually be able to move the affected limb and even use it to a certain extent the child with a broken bone will probably not be able to use the limb at all.

What types of fracture are there?

A simple fracture is one in which the bones have not broken through the skin. A compound or open fracture is one in which the bones have broken through the skin. (In a compound fracture there is an added risk of the wound becoming infected.)

In a comminuted fracture the bone is broken into several pieces.

In an undisplaced fracture the two ends of broken bone are still in contact with one another.

In a displaced fracture the two ends of broken bone are not in contact with one another and may need to be realigned before the bone can set again.

In a complicated fracture the bone has damaged a nerve or blood vessel.

In an impacted fracture the two ends of broken bone are pushed into each other like two cars fixed together after an accident.

A bone is said to be chipped when a small piece has been broken off.

Fractures are also sometimes described as splintered, transverse, oblique and spiral. These terms are self-explanatory.

In a greenstick fracture there is no genuine break but the bone has actually bent – rather like a piece of green stick.

What can we do about it?

If you think there is any chance that your child has fractured a bone then you should get medical help straight away. You should not try to push any protruding bone back into place, you should not try to clean out a wound yourself, you should not move the child any more than is absolutely necessary in order to avoid further danger (and then you should move the child in such a way that he is not bent or twisted in any additional way) and you should not let the child move the affected part. If you use a splint adjust the splint to fit the limb rather than the other way round.

If the affected bone is an arm you can take the child to the nearest hospital yourself but if the suspected break involves the neck or backbone then you should not move the patient at all. Moving a child with a broken back can damage the spinal nerves and produce a permanent paralysis. If the accident has happened on the road use motor cars and hazard flashers to act as a screen and warning sign for approaching traffic and wait until an ambulance arrives before moving the victim.

A child with a suspected fracture should have nothing to eat or drink in case an operation is necessary.

What's the difference between a fracture and a dislocation?
A dislocation involves a joint and no broken bones. A dislocated joint will be very painful, will look deformed and will be immovable. It is important not to try and put a dislocated joint back into position unless you know what you are doing. You should try and keep the patient as comfortable as possible while you wait for expert medical help to arrive.

Will a fractured limb lead to a deformity?
Most fractures heal well. This is particularly true of children, whose bones are capable not only of healing but also of correcting any abnormality that may remain after a fracture. Children's bones are growing bones and they are able to repair themselves very effectively. Fractures which occur near the ends of long bones (such as the femur in the leg) can cause problems since they may affect the growth of the bone.

Bones heal quicker in children than in adults.

How can we make a splint for a broken bone?
Splints are useful because they help immobilise damaged limbs. They can be made from wood, metal, umbrellas, stiffly rolled newspapers or healthy limbs. The splint should be bound to the limb above and below the break but care should be taken not to fasten the splint too tightly since this could impede the circulation of the blood.

When do we need to see a doctor?
You need medical advice about any possible fracture. If you are

not certain about the nature of any damage that may have been done then you need a doctor's advice. If the limb is not obviously broken your family doctor is the best person to consult since he will be able to tell you whether or not an X-ray is required. If the limb is obviously broken then the child will almost certainly need hospital treatment.

What will the doctor do?

If he thinks that there is any chance that a bone could be broken your doctor will arrange for an X-ray to be taken. An X-ray shows up the bones clearly and will enable the doctors to decide whether or not there is a fracture and, if there is, what sort of fracture it is.

Once a fracture has been diagnosed the treatment will depend upon the site and the type of fracture. Whatever is decided pain relief will obviously be a priority.

If the fracture has broken the skin then the wound will have to be cleaned very carefully and tetanus protection will be required. If the bones are undisplaced the doctors may not need to do anything but immobilise the limb either with a splint or a cast made out of plaster of paris. If the bones are displaced then the bones will need to be set and fixed in place. In some circumstances bones will need to be fixed together with metal pins so that they can heal properly. These pins may need to be removed at some later stage.

Bones take some time to knit together properly and a major break may need six to ten weeks to heal properly. Smaller breaks in smaller bones may take less than that.

Burns and scalds

What causes them?

Burns are skin injuries which can usually be put into one of three main categories. They are either dry burns caused by fire, by electricity, by friction or by contact with a piece of hot material; they are chemical burns caused by acids, alkalis or other strong chemicals; or they are scalds caused by very hot liquids or fat.

What types of burn are there?

Burns are classified according to the depth and extent to which they have damaged the skin. Superficial or first-degree burns simply cause reddening of the skin and some pain. These burns don't usually cause any scarring. Second-degree burns always cause blistering of the skin in addition to the reddening. The blisters are caused by fluid leaking out of the blood vessels damaged inside the tissues. Third-degree burns are the deepest and most serious and they involve the death of a full layer of skin. The skin in a third-degree burn will either be blackened or will be white.

When are burns dangerous?

Any third-degree burn, however small it is, is potentially dangerous since it can result in infection and scarring. First-degree burns are less commonly serious. Second-degree burns are serious and dangerous if they involve more than 10 per cent of the skin's surface area.

Any burn which involves the face, the joints or the hands is particularly dangerous since the resultant scarring can be either disfiguring or disabling. And any burn which is also associated with a loss of body fluids can be dangerous since the fluid loss can produce shock. It is important to remember that pain is not a useful guide to a burn's seriousness. Very severe burns can destroy nerve endings with the result that no pain is felt.

What can we do about burns?

1 Immerse the burnt area in cold water. If the burn can be dipped into the sink or a bowl then that will do fine. If the burnt area involves too much skin for the sink then use a bath. This simple first aid measure may be painful but it will help prevent blistering and will minimise the amount of damage done to the tissues. A burn should be kept immersed for at least ten minutes.
2 If the burn is a second- or third-degree burn then you should seek medical advice straight away.
3 If the burn is a second-degree burn and there has to be some delay before you obtain medical advice then you can put a clean dry dressing on to it. Don't use any material which is likely to leave bits of cloth sticking to the skin.
4 If the burn is on a finger or hand remove all rings and bracelets. The tissues may well swell and if they do those rings and bracelets may cause problems.

What shouldn't we do about burns?

1 Don't put butter on to a burn. And don't put any other type of cream or ointment on either. Butter won't help at all and it may, indeed, make things considerably worse by turning the burnt area into a sticky mess.

2 Don't try picking off any bits of burnt clothing. You may do more harm than good if you try doing this yourself.

3 Try not to touch the burnt area any more than you have to and try not to breathe on it either.

4 Don't burst blisters.

What will the doctor do?

Your doctor will either provide first aid advice or, if he considers that the burn is too serious to be allowed to repair itself at home, he will arrange emergency hospital admission. Children with third-degree burns will usually be admitted to hospital as will children with second-degree burns that cover more than 10 per cent of the skin, and children with second-degree burns that affect the face, hands or joints.

In hospital attention will be paid to dressing the burns carefully so as to minimise the risk of infection. The doctors will also replace fluid lost through the burnt area of skin.

Once the emergency situation has been put under control the doctors will decide how best to cope with the damaged area of skin. Skin grafting, using either a very thin layer of the patient's own skin taken from another part of his body or a piece of skin from a 'skin bank' will often be very effective in minimising the resultant scarring.

How can we prevent burns?

Burns are one of the major causes of death among young children and a major cause of many serious accidents. Most burns could have been prevented with a little care. I've compiled a list of precautions for parents to take.

1 Don't let children jump into the bath or shower without first testing the water. If you have a shower that isn't thermostatically controlled and able to maintain its own temperature independently of other water supplies in the house take care to insist that no one turns on any tap while a child is using the shower.

2 Teach your children to be aware of the risks associated with fires and electrical appliances.

3 Keep open fires guarded.

4 Try and ensure that your children wear non-inflammable night clothes.

5 Check your electrical appliances regularly to make sure that wires are not getting frayed. Children sometimes chew on extension leads and serious electrical burns can occur this way.

6 Do not keep gasoline or any other inflammable materials in your home.

7 Keep chemicals, such as bleach and powerful disinfectants, well out of reach, preferably in locked cupboards.

8 Keep matches, lighters and so on out of reach.

9 Turn pan handles inwards when they are on the stove to prevent small children reaching up and pulling pans down on top of them. This is still a common cause of severe scalds.

10 A large number of burns occur because the ordinary hot water in the house is heated to too high a temperature. Hot water in your house shouldn't be higher than 120 degrees Fahrenheit or about 50 degrees centigrade.

Catarrh

What is it?

The nose, and the series of passageways and cavities which connect it to the throat, are lined with a thin layer of tissue equipped with many tiny mucus-producing glands. Known as the mucous membrane, this lining is kept moist by the secretions produced by the glands.

Under normal circumstances these secretions help to keep the passageways clean and they prevent the steady flow of air from drying the tissues too much.

If the mucous membranes become inflamed for any reason they may be stimulated to overproduce mucus. And catarrh is simply the result of mucous membranes producing too much mucus.

What cause it?

Two things can inflame the membranes: infections and allergies. The common cold is probably the most frequent type of infection responsible but infections of the sinuses and the chest can also be associated with catarrh. Allergies such as hay fever also irritate the mucous membranes and stimulate them to over-produce mucus. Seasonal catarrh is often caused by an allergy.

How do we make the diagnosis?
The excessive secretions can cause stuffiness and can build up to cause headaches which are usually confined to the front part of the head. Secretions dripping down the back of the throat can cause coughing which will keep the child awake at night. Children may swallow catarrh if they cannot cough it up and that may make them vomit.

Is it catching?
Infections which cause catarrh may be catching but catarrh is not.

What can we do about it?
If the catarrh is caused by an allergy the problem won't be solved until contact with the allergen has been broken (see also page 22). Antihistamines may alleviate the symptoms.

Symptoms in older children can often be alleviated by a simple menthol inhalation which will help clear the sinuses and relieve stuffiness, headaches and coughing. A small menthol crystal or a smear of a menthol rub is put into a bowl and hot water is added. The child is then encouraged to breathe in the rising vapour. Younger children who cannot manage an inhalation will some-times get relief if a kettle is boiled in the room in which they are sleeping. The extra moisture in the air helps clear away the sticky, mucous secretions.

To minimise symptoms make sure that no one smokes in the same room as the patient since cigarette smoke can make things worse. For mild headaches use paracetamol or aspirin.

I do not recommend the use of any decongestants or nasal sprays. These may produce temporary relief but when they are not used the congestion and catarrh will often return. The end result may be that the condition is made worse by the treatment.

When do we need to see the doctor?
If symptoms persist for more than five days, recur or cause distress which you cannot relieve.

Chest pain

What is it?
This is a common problem among children. In adults chest pain is often a serious symptom – in children it is usually of little significance.

What causes it?
Most children will usually suffer what are called 'stitch' pains after exercising fiercely. These pains usually occur in the lower part of the chest and are more common on the left side than the right. No one really seems to know what causes 'stitch' pains but the explanations include spasm of the diaphragm, contraction of the spleen and gas in the intestines. Whatever the cause these strange pains seem to disappear after a few moments' rest.

Coughing often causes pain in the centre of the chest and may in addition cause pain in the ribs. Vomiting can also cause rib pains.

Injuries cause the majority of other pains in the chest with bruises, muscle strains and cracked ribs all being fairly insignificant in harsh clinical terms even though they may seem to cause a considerable amount of discomfort.

The serious causes of chest pain in children are limited in number and extremely uncommon. Heart pains are more or less unknown but occasionally severe chest infections or lung problems can cause pain. These problems are usually associated with breathlessness.

What can we do about it?
Obviously the treatment depends on the cause and the extent of the pain.

When do we need to see the doctor?
If a chest pain is accompanied by breathlessness or is not relieved with the aid of mild painkillers (such as aspirin, paracetemol and a hot-water bottle), a doctor's advice should be sought.

What will the doctor do?
The doctor will be able to examine the child's chest and exclude any of the serious and rare disorders which need medical

attention. He will probably not provide any treatment for most cases of chest pain. Today few doctors believe that strapping fractured ribs helps speed healing or relieve pain.

Chickenpox

What is it?
A very common infectious disease caused by a virus.

How do we make the diagnosis?
To begin with the spots look like small pimples. Then in a day or so they gradually grow into blisters which obviously contain fluid. The spots can start just about anywhere on the body but usually seem to begin on the head. They can occur inside the mouth where they are particularly painful. The chest and abdomen tend to be more severely affected than the arms and legs. Chickenpox spots continue to arrive for three our four days; this means that at any one time there will be spots present in several stages of development. It's rarely possible to make a diagnosis before the spots become clearly visible although just before the character-istic rash appears the child will usually complain of a headache and may have a fever and an indistinct blotchy rash.

Is it catching?
Chickenpox is very infectious. It is spread by touch or breath. After contact with an infected individual a child may take two to three weeks to produce symptoms. A child with chickenpox is infectious from twenty-four hours before the spots appear until the spots have all turned into dried scabs. The scabs are not infectious.

What can we do about it?
There is no cure for chickenpox. The commonest symptom associated with the disease is itching and this can often be best dealt with by an application of calamine lotion. If the patient scratches too much permanent scars can ensue so it is important to alleviate itching as much as possible. The damage done by night-time scratching can be minimised by getting the child to wear gloves or mittens.

Is there a link with shingles?

Chickenpox and shingles are caused by the same virus or by very similar viruses. The precise relationship between the two disorders is still a subject of considerable debate but it does seem possible for children to catch chickenpox from adults with shingles.

When do we need to see the doctor?

If the itching is very bad there is a risk that the spots will become infected. So if calamine doesn't help ask your doctor for assistance. He may, for example, prescribe an antihistamine to help dampen down the need to scratch.

A child who has obviously got chickenpox should be quite well apart from his itchy rash. If there are other symptoms it is important to get in touch with the doctor since there can occasionally be complications. Vomiting, headaches and sleepiness are three of the most important to watch out for.

Choking

What is it?

Choking is caused by a genuine inability to breathe. A child who is choking will be frantically struggling to breathe and will be unable to cry out or speak. Choking is a genuine emergency since it can kill. Within a minute or two the choking child will turn blue, convulse, go limp and become unconscious.

How do we make the diagnosis?

There isn't usually any difficulty in making the diagnosis. When a child is deliberately breath holding he won't be trying to breathe. During a convulsion when a child's breathing may be erratic he will often cry out and there will be no tremendous effort to breathe. In gagging, caused by an irritation to the throat, there will only be momentary interference with breathing.

What causes it?

Choking is the result of a blockage in the pipe which carries air down into the lungs. This can occasionally be caused by severe infections of the chest but is most commonly caused by some foreign object getting stuck or 'going down the wrong way'.

Sweets, small toys, beads and pieces of food are common causes of choking. Eating when walking about or running is a common cause of choking and small sweets and peanuts are the commonest culprits.

What can we do about it?

Choking is a genuine emergency and it must be dealt with as quickly as possible.

If the choking victim is a baby or very small child hold him up upside down by the legs and smack him hard on the back until the object has been dislodged. A tap won't do, you really must slap quite hard. Don't worry about bruising or even breaking ribs. If you don't get that object out of his windpipe he will die.

If the victim is a larger child you can either put him over your knee with his head down near the floor and smack him hard on his back or you can try the Heimlich manoeuvre. To do this stand behind the child, put your arms around him with your hands clenched together over the upper part of his abdomen and then press suddenly and upwards. By compressing the upper abdomen you will push the diaphragm up so quickly that air in the lungs will force the object causing the obstruction out of the airway.

While you are trying one of these procedures scream for help and get someone to telephone for an ambulance and a doctor.

Once you think you've got the foreign object into the throat or mouth you can use your fingers to hook it out if it doesn't pop out of its own accord. Do be careful not to push it further in.

Don't try the kiss of life if a child inhales an object because you may blow the foreign object further into the lungs and make it even more difficult to remove. Once you've removed the object c⌐ ⌐he blockage you can try mouth-to-mouth resuscitation if ⌐ill not breathing.

⌐ advice?

U⌐ ⌐he obstruction is complete you w⌐ ⌐ yourself or else it will be too ⌐ ⌐ be complete and even if you⌐ ⌐ill seek medical help as urgently ⌐ the object by any of the metho⌐

How can we prevent choking?

1 Don't let babies and small children eat peanuts or tiny sweets.

2 Don't let children eat while they are walking or running about.

3 Make sure that toys small children play with are too large to put into the mouth. Beads and glass eyes from stuffed animals commonly cause choking.

4 Don't let children play games in which they throw sweets or peanuts into the air and then catch them in their mouths.

5 A child who is vomiting should lie on his side or his front but not on his back.

Circumcision

What is it?

The end of the male organ or penis is, at birth, covered with a loose fold of skin known as the foreskin. The removal of this fold of skin for any reason is known as circumcision.

Why is it done?

Circumcision is carried out for a number of reasons. Male members of the Muslim and Jewish religion are, for example, routinely circumcised purely to satisfy the demands of their religion. In some parts of the world circumcision is carried out fairly routinely because doctors believe that circumcision is an essential aid to hygiene. And, of course, circumcision is also carried out if the foreskin is so tight that it cannot be retracted and it impedes the passage of urine.

When is circumcision essential?

The foreskin is attached to the end of the penis in the newborn male and it isn't until the age of 3 or 4 years that the foreskin can be fully retracted. It is therefore important to realise that circumcision is not always essential simply because the foreskin cannot be retracted. (The medical term for this is phimosis.)

Circumcision is essential if:

1 There is no opening in the foreskin.

2 The opening is too small to allow urine to pass through. If this is the case the foreskin will always 'balloon' when the child tries to pass urine. This condition is in fact quite rare.

3 There are recurrent infections on and around the end of the penis.

4 A paraphimosis develops. In this condition the foreskin becomes permanently and painfully retracted.

5 If a boy of 5 years or over cannot retract his foreskin at all then some form of surgical advice may be required. In some circumstances a circumcision may not be necessary and the surgeon may be able simply to free the foreskin. A researcher who made observations of 9,545 Copenhagen schoolboys showed that although 8 per cent couldn't retract their foreskins at the age of 6 or 7 years only 1 per cent had the same problem ten years later.

Does circumcision contribute to the standard of male hygiene?
No. A foreskin that can be fully retracted can be kept clean and free from infection quite easily. Circumcision is not, therefore, an essential aid to hygiene.

What about if the foreskin is too long?
It won't be.

What are the advantages of circumcision?
1 It is said by some doctors that men who are circumcised will have a reduced chance of developing cancer of the penis. This condition is extremely rare and I don't know of any convincing evidence which supports this claim.

2 It is also claimed that the female partners of circumcised men are less likely to develop cervical cancer. This may be true where circumcised males are compared with uncircumcised males with low standards of personal hygiene.

3 Removal of the foreskin leads to a decreased sensitivity of the glans penis. This is turn delays ejaculation. This can be an advantage in men who suffer from premature ejaculation. Since there is no way of knowing whether your child is going to suffer from premature ejaculation or is going to have difficulty in reaching ejaculation there is no way of knowing whether or not he (and his partners) will consider his circumcision an advantage or a disadvantage.

4 When the foreskin has been removed there is no risk of paraphimosis developing. (This is a painful condition in which the foreskin becomes irreversibly retracted and tightens around the penis.)

What are the disadvantages of circumcision?

1 A circumcision is an operation, albeit a small one. There are therefore the inevitable risks associated with any form of operation. A small number of boys die.

2 If the circumcision is performed without a high degree of skill there may be damage done to the penis. Bleeding and post-operative infection are not unknown.

3 Scarring is sometimes considered unsightly.

4 The decreased sensitivity of the glans penis is considered a disadvantage by some individuals.

Should we have our son circumcised?

I do not presume to offer advice to parents who want to have their sons circumcised on religious grounds, although I would just make the point that to have the operation done without an anaesthetic is barbaric and inhumane. If such an operation were performed on animals who had not been anaesthetised there would be a public outcry.

If there are no religious reasons for circumcision and there are no acute medical problems for which circumcision is the only recommended remedy you should discuss the question with your own family doctor. My advice is not to have your son circumcised.

What about girls?

I should mention, I suppose, that in some parts of the world girls are circumcised with the foreskin of the clitoris being removed. There are never any medical reasons for this operation which is only ever performed for religious, social or sexual reasons.

Cleft palate

What is it?

In a child with a cleft palate the hard roof of the mouth is improperly formed with a gap being left in the middle where the two sides of the palate have failed to come together. A cleft palate may or may not be associated with a cleft or hare lip in which the upper lip also has a gap in the middle.

Cleft lip is slightly more common than cleft palate.

What causes it?

Both these problems are a result of a development problem in the womb. The direct cause has not yet been identified although a number of possible causes have been suggested. The condition can be inherited.

How do we make the diagnosis?

The diagnosis is obviously easy to make when the problem affects the lip. When only the palate is involved mothers may only realise that something is wrong when they notice that their baby is having difficulty in sucking.

What can we do about it?

If the baby with a cleft palate has real difficulty in sucking it may be advisable to feed the baby with a spoon. It is, however, of prime importance to seek medical advice as soon as possible, whether the condition affects the upper lip alone, the palate alone, or both together.

What will the doctor do?

The first thing your doctor should do is offer support, encouragement and hope. Parents are always worried by cleft palates and hare lips but modern surgical techniques are extremely effective at repairing these faults.

Cleft lips can usually be repaired within a few months of birth but operations to repair cleft palates are sometimes left rather later than this. Until the palate is repaired, however, it is usual to provide a special prosthesis; this will make feeding far easier.

Will our child be able to speak without impediment?

The majority of children who have cleft palates end up speaking quite clearly. Where there are problems in speaking advice and help from speech therapists will usually be provided.

Will our child need plastic surgery?

If after the cleft lip or palate have been repaired there are still signs of the original abnormality or, indeed, signs of any imperfection, advice from a plastic surgeon should be sought. If any residual imperfection involves the teeth then advice from an orthodontic specialist should be sought.

Colic

What is it?
Strictly speaking the word 'colic' means any cramp-like intermittent abdominal pain. But the word is most widely used to describe the severe abdominal pain that commonly affects babies between two weeks and three months of age. Because it tends to go on for three months and then disappear colic is sometimes known as 'three months colic'. It often seems to occur in the early evening, may last up to four hours at a time, and seems to affect between 10 and 20 per cent of babies.

The baby with colic usually cries continually, clenches his fists, pulls his legs up, screams and goes quite red. This can go on for day after day, beginning in the late afternoon and going on all through the evening.

What causes it?
I don't think anyone really knows what causes colic although a number of doctors have come up with explanations. Some say that gas causes colic and that it is the gas building up inside the gut which causes the pain. Others claim that there is some ingredient in cows' milk which causes colic. In support of their theory these researchers have done work which shows that breast fed children are less likely to get colic and that there is a protein in cows' milk to which babies can become sensitive.

How do we make the diagnosis?
It is by no means easy to diagnose colic with any degree of certainty and it is dangerous to assume that a baby has colic unless other possible causes have been excluded.

If your baby is in pain and you are not certain that it is caused by colic you should ask for medical advice. Other possible causes of abdominal pain must be ruled out before the diagnosis of colic is made. It is also essential to exclude other causes of discomfort such as constipation, diarrhoea, nappy rash and infections.

What can we do about it?

If your baby has persistent colicky pains which you are certain are not caused by any more serious disorder which requires medical attention try picking him up and feeding him. If your baby takes the offered food and then sleeps happily then he was hungry, not suffering from colic. If you are breast feeding do make sure that your nipples are not bleeding since swallowed blood can cause cramps.

If the crying stops when the baby is picked up then the chances are that the baby was simply lonely or bored and wanted some company. Again, it is unlikely that the cause was colic.

There is no real evidence that colic is caused by excessive wind but it's probably worthwhile trying to avoid allowing your baby to acquire too much wind. To do this try and make sure that your baby doesn't swallow air when he is feeding and burp him carefully after the feeding.

Try and remain as calm as possible while your baby is crying with what you assume is colic. Some doctors have suggested that what we describe as colic is in fact caused by the baby being aware that mum is getting harassed. They claim that a baby whose mother is quiet and relaxed will suffer far less from colic.

There are many gripe waters and mixtures about which are sold to help colicky babies. I don't recommend any of these but you can try one of the medicines containing dicyclomine hydrochloride which does seem to be remarkably efficient at banishing the problem. A little gentle warmth as applied with the aid of a hot-water bottle also seems to help.

When to see the doctor?

You should seek medical advice if your baby is off his feeds, if he has diarrhoea, if he vomits and if he goes very quiet or pale. You should also seek medical advice if your baby cries persistently and you are not satisfied that the cause is colic.

Common cold

What is it?

A viral infection that affects most children at least three times a year.

How do we make the diagnosis?

The early symptoms of a cold are usually a sore throat and a tendency to sniff and sneeze frequently. Sufferers sometimes complain of a slight general aching, a headache and a fever. The symptoms of a cold are rarely severe and are usually more inconvenient than incapacitating, annoying rather than disabling.

Is it infectious?

A good deal of research has been done in an attempt to discover just how the common cold is transmitted from one sufferer to another. It used to be thought that it was possible to catch a cold by going out of doors with wet hair or by standing around with wet feet. Another common myth is that colds occur more frequently in the cold weather.

The truth seems to be that there is not any real relationship between the cold weather and colds. Nor is there any connection between colds and dampness.

Until quite recently it was also believed that most colds were passed on in droplets and that standing in the way of a sneeze was the best way to catch a cold. This is now not believed to be the case. Researchers suggest that most colds are transmitted by touch and that the cold virus gets into the human body through the nose or the tear ducts. The virus arrives there on the potential sufferer's own hands.

This new evidence suggests that the best way to help children avoid catching colds is to persuade them to try and touch their faces as infrequently as possible.

You may not think that your child touches his or her face very often but if you sit and watch for a minute or two you'll soon see just how often the hands do touch the nose and eyes.

What can we do about it?

There is no cure for the common cold and there is no vaccine yet available which will provide any protection. There is no vaccine simply because there are something like 200 different cold-producing viruses and no one vaccine could do more than provide protection against one of those viruses.

Nor, I'm afraid, is there any convincing evidence to suggest that vitamin C supplements or any other tonic will prevent colds developing. It is quite true that a child who has been living on a diet deficient in vitamin C will be more susceptible to the cold viruses. But a child who has been fed properly and who has an adequate intake of vitamin C will not benefit from having an extra dose. Vitamin C is a water-soluble vitamin and once the body has acquired the amount of vitamin C it needs it excretes any excess in the urine.

Soluble aspirin tablets or paracetamol medicine given according to the manufacturer's instructions will relieve the aching and will help reduce any fever. There isn't any other really effective way to deal with the general symptoms of a cold.

The runny nose and the stuffiness are common problems, of course, and there are a number of special preparations available over the counter which are intended to deal with these two symptoms.

I don't recommend any of these products for several reasons. The first is that the drugs which are used to help dry up secretions and the drugs which are used to help clear congestion can call produce problems of their own. The second is that they do, on the whole, only offer a temporary respite. You may be able to stop the runny nose by using a branded medicine but there is a good chance that as soon as you stop using the medicine the symptoms will recur. If a child has to attend some important event, such as a special party or a school concert, it may be worthwhile trying one of the multipurpose cold remedies, but I don't recommend that you use them for anything more than a temporary effect.

The stuffed-up feeling that children often get with a cold is best relieved with a good old-fashioned inhalation. Just pour some hot water into a bowl, add a menthol crystal and let your young patient breathe in the medicated steam as it rises. Put a towel over his head if you like to help keep the vapour in the right place. Younger children who cannot be helped in this way will feel better if you simply boil the kettle and let the vapour fill the air. You can help relieve the stuffed-up feeling that keeps children awake by putting a small dab of a mentholated balm on to the child's chest.

The only other general piece of advice I can offer is that you make up a hot lemon drink. Slice five lemons into two pints of cold water and add two tablespoonfuls of sugar or honey. Bring it all to the boil and simmer, reducing the liquid slightly. Then allow it all to cool. Afterwards add hot water to the concentrate as and when you need it. If you serve it in a large glass and persuade the child to sniff the rising fumes you can use the drink as an inhalant and a soothing remedy for an irritated throat.

If your child also has a cough or a sore throat then see pages 94 and 216 respectively.

How can we differentiate between colds and flu?

The child who has flu will obviously be ill whereas the child who has a cold will simply be miserable. The child who is too ill and unhappy to eat, read, play or watch the television is more likely to have flu (or some other disorder) than a simple cold and he needs to be seen by a doctor.

Generally speaking the patient with a cold will complain mainly of a streaming nose and of sneezing attacks whereas the patient with flu will sweat a good deal and will be very weak. Muscle aches and pains are also more common and more severe with flu and they may make walking and moving about quite difficult.

What other diseases can mimic a cold?

The early symptoms of a common cold are similar to the early symptoms of other diseases – notably measles and german measles. The rashes associated with these infections will usually become quite apparent within a day or two.

When do we need to see the doctor?

If your child simply has a cold then no doctor can help you. Antibiotics and other similar drugs such as penicillin are useless for treating the ordinary cold since they only affect bacteria and colds are produced by viruses. Your doctor can only suggest that you use such well-established standards as aspirin or paracetamol.

However, if you suspect that your child's cold has developed into something else or if you feel that he might have flu then you should get in touch. A cold will not normally last more than seven days and there will usually be genuine signs of improvement within five days.

A child who is coughing a good deal, vomiting or not eating is likely to have something more serious than a common cold and may, therefore, need to see a doctor.

Any child who wants to stay in bed and won't even get up to watch television is ill enough to need medical attention.

Congenital problems

What are they?
Each human baby that is born grows from the union of a single spermatozoa and a single egg. If there is any genetic abnormality or if the development process is in any way interrupted then the foetus which develops may be in some way abnormal. The nature and extent of the deformity can vary a great deal from the trivial and relatively insignificant to the serious and life-threatening. In the most severe instances the foetus is likely to be aborted at an early stage.

Out of a hundred babies three or four will show some signs of abnormality. The more significant abnormalities include congenital dislocation of the hip (in which a baby is born with a malformed hip joint), congenital heart abnormalities (there are many different types of problem within this general category), and cleft palate. Less significant abnormalities include webbing between the fingers, extra toes and birthmarks.

What causes them?
1 Many congenital problems are inherited. Each human baby grows from a mixture of chromosomes provided by both parents. Those chromosomes carry blueprints for the production of the baby. The genes can carry good points but they can also carry bad points too. If your parents were both tall and good-looking then you've got a better than average chance of being tall and good-looking. Similarly if your parents both had asthma then you've got a better than average change of developing asthma.
2 Infections which affect the pregnant mother, and thereby her unborn child, can cause congenital abnormalities. The best known infection to produce problems is perhaps rubella or german measles. If a woman is infected during the first three months of pregnancy she may have a miscarriage but if the baby survives it may be born blind, deaf or with a heart disorder. Some babies have all these problems. Mental retardation is another problem associated with the rubella infection.
3 Since the thalidomide disaster it has been well known that many drugs can damage the foetus if taken by a pregnant woman. Thalidomide produced a condition known as phocomelia in which the limbs failed to develop properly.
4 Diagnostic tools can produce a wide variety of problems. If X-

rays are used to excess on a developing foetus then damage can be done to the ovaries or testes of that foetus with possible ill effect on the subsequent generation.

5 There are, in addition, a number of other factors which influence the incidence of congenital abnormalities. Although we still have much to learn it seems that the types of food eaten, the purity of the water drunk, the age of the parents and countless other variations can all have an influence.

What will the doctor do about it?

Babies are routinely examined just after birth in order to look for any signs of abnormality. Any abnormalities which are identified will be treated appropriately without delay. Some congenital disorders (pyloric stenosis and congenital dislocation of the hip, for example) can be permanently cured surgically.

Conjunctivitis

What is it?

The thin and sensitive membrane that covers the surface of the eye is called the conjunctiva. If this membrane becomes irritated the condition is known as 'conjunctivitis'.

What causes it?

The usual cause of conjunctivitis is an infection although foreign bodies that get into the eye and irritate it can cause an inflammation of the conjunctiva as can products which trigger off allergy reactions.

How can we make the diagnosis?

It is important to be able to differentiate between the various possible causes of conjunctivitis in order to deal effectively with the source of the problem.

When conjunctivitis is due to an allergy reaction (either because the eye has been in close contact with some substance such as a cosmetic or because of some more general problem such as hay fever) then the symptoms will usually be confined to itching, watering and redness. There is often some swelling around the eye.

When the conjunctivitis is due to an infection the eye will

usually be sticky with the patient complaining of a 'grittiness'. This feeling is usually worse first thing in the morning and patients will often complain that they feel as though they have something in their eyes. When an infection has caused the conjunctivitis there is often a yellow discharge of pus that collects most obviously in the corner of the affected eye. The pus collects during the night and is therefore most easily seen first thing in the morning. As a result of the accumulation of this sticky discharge the eyelids are often stuck together – sometimes needing to be prised apart.

Differentiating between the various non-infective causes of conjunctivitis is often just a matter of common sense. When a child is known to suffer from hay fever and he complains of itchy eyes during the hay fever season the probable diagnosis isn't difficult to make. When a young girl has been experimenting with her mother's eye make-up and she subsequently develops sore, itchy eyes then the problem is likely to be a specific allergy reaction.

What is a 'sticky eye'?
This term is sometimes used to describe all forms of conjunctivitis in which the lids are glued together. Usually, however, it is reserved for those cases of conjunctivitis which affect newborn babies. 'Sticky eye' in small babies is usually produced by debris accumulating in and around the eye at birth.

Is conjunctivitis infectious?
Conjunctivitis caused by a local infection of the conjunctiva is very infectious and care should be taken to ensure that the infection is not spread from one child to another. Encourage children not to rub their eyes and to wash and dry their hands and faces with disposable towels. Conjunctivitis can be spread from one of a child's eyes to the other eye. The incubation period is usually less than three days.

Conjunctivitis produced by causes other than infection is not contagious.

Does conjunctivitis always affect both eyes?
No. If the conjunctivitis is caused by an infection then it won't affect both eyes unless the infection spreads from one eye to the other. If the conjunctivitis is caused by an allergic reaction then it

will only affect both eyes if both eyes have been exposed to the allergen. However, some doctors do suggest that if you are treating one eye for an infected conjunctivitis you should also treat the other eye with the same remedy in order to prevent the infection from spreading.

What can we do about it?

If you are convinced that the conjunctivitis is a result of some non-infectious problem then the solution will be fairly straight-forward. If you suspect that the conjunctivitis has been caused by some localised allergy reaction then you must first try and decide what the problem substance is and then try to ensure that future contact is prevented. If you suspect that your child's conjunctivitis is a result of a more generalised allergy reaction then the most appropriate treatment will obviously be directed towards solving that particular problem rather than simply trying to deal with the conjunctivitis. So, for example, if you suspect that your child's sore and itchy eyes are associated with his hay fever then the most appropriate treatment will be treatment designed to deal with the hay fever.

Should you feel that your child's conjunctivitis has been caused by an infection then you must seek medical advice as soon as possible since the only real answer is to use antibiotic drops or ointment. While waiting for medical prescribed treatment you can ease the symptoms in several ways.

If your child's eyelids are stuck together then you will probably be able to part them by bathing with a warm, clean sponge or face cloth. Do make sure that you clean the sponge thoroughly afterwards for eye infections can easily spread.

Many children are bothered by the light when they have conjunctivitis and these can usually be helped by being given dark glasses to wear. Alternatively, of course, they will probably be comfortable if you can keep the curtains closed and the sunlight temporarily shut out.

When should we see the doctor?

You should see the doctor straight away if your child is complaining of any loss of vision, whether it be temporary or apparently permanent, partial or total, or if your child is complaining of actual pain in or around his eye. Children with conjunctivitis will complain of soreness and 'grittiness' but they will not usually complain of any actual pain.

You should also see your doctor if you suspect that your child could have any foreign body in his eye. Even if you cannot actually see anything in the eye you should remember that tiny flies and very small specks of dust can sometimes remain almost invisible while producing quite insignificant symptoms. If your child has been doing anything which may have resulted in a foreign object getting into the eye then ask your doctor to make the appropriate examination. Some doctors may not have the equipment needed for this type of examination and may prefer you to visit the local casualty department. It is probably sensible to telephone first for advice.

Cycling downhill seems to be a very good way to get flies and specks of dust into the eyes, by the way!

If your child has a conjunctivitis that you suspect is or may be infectious in origin then you should make an appointment for a consultation as soon as possible since the only appropriate treatment is to use an antibiotic ointment or some antibiotic drops.

If you are convinced that your child's eye symptoms are the result of some other problem – such as an allergy reaction – and you think that you can deal with it effectively either by coping with the source of the allergy or by providing some form of treatment then you should still seek medical advice if the symptoms last for more than an additional twenty-four hours.

Conjunctivitis sometimes accompanies other diseases – particularly measles. You should, therefore, keep an eye out for rashes and call for medical advice if you think you need it.

What will the doctor do?

Some doctors will take swabs from children's eyes in order to isolate and identify the organism which has produced the infection. Others will decide to treat the infection straight away with an antibiotic. If he is looking for a foreign body or a sign of any damage to the eye your doctor may temporarily stain the eyeball with special drops.

Doctors sometimes ask parents whether they prefer ointment or drops. There is rarely any genuine medical reason to prefer one to the other. Many parents seem to find ointment easier than drops since drops usually find their way everywhere except into the patient's eyes. Whichever form of treatment is eventually selected it is important to ensure that the course of treatment is completed (this will usually last for five days or so) and that any residue is thrown away. Ointments and drops intended for use in the eyes deteriorate quite quickly once they have been opened and should certainly not be kept in the bathroom cabinet for some future occasion.

If your doctor is himself uncertain about the diagnosis or the most appropriate treatment he will usually arrange for immediate referral to an ophthalmologist.

Constipation

What is it?
The incidence of constipation among babies and young children is far less common than many mothers might suppose for whereas many mothers regard the frequency of bowel movement as being the most vital factor it is the nature of the consistency of the stool which is much more important.

There is a tradition that if bowels are not opened and emptied as regularly as post boxes then there is something wrong. Thousands of tiny bowels are attacked daily with powerful laxatives by mothers who believe this nonsense.

The frequency with which the bowels are opened is of no significance as far as most babies and young children are concerned. Just because nothing is passed for a day or two or even for a week it doesn't mean that the child is constipated. Much more important is the nature and consistency of the stool that is passed. Small, hard stools that can only be passed with difficulty, discomfort and great effort are good solid evidence of constipation.

That simple rule is good for babies, toddlers and children of all ages.

What causes it?
The single most important cause of constipation involves the diet. With human beings, as with anything else, you only get out what you put in. The relationship to diet is particularly true for babies. Constipation is extremely rare among breast fed babies. Breast milk was formulated by the best expert there is and contains very little waste. Consequently a breast fed baby can happily go a

week without a bowel movement. Among bottle fed babies
constipation is rather more common. Using too much milk
powder is the most common cause.

What can we do about it?

When bottle fed babies are constipated the problem can usually
be alleviated by adding a little brown sugar to the feed, adding
more water or including a feed of fruit juice at some time during
the day. If those simple solutions don't work then it is worth
considering the possibility that the baby might have been
underfed.

Diet is also a common cause of constipation among toddlers. To
help cope with the problem I would recommend plenty of fluids,
lots of fruit (apart from bananas), a good supply of fresh fruit juice,
wholemeal bread, cereals, bran, brown sugar, honey and green
vegetables. Remember that milk, biscuits, sweets and cake all
make constipation worse. In addition, do remember that toddlers
sometimes get constipated because they are under so much
pressure from their parents to perform regularly and effectively
that they rebel and refuse to perform. When that happens the
best remedy is to leave things along for a while and to withdraw
the pressure.

When constipation occurs in older children it may sometimes
be a result of shyness or embarrassment. Children get constipated because they find school lavatories cold, dirty, smelly or
lacking in privacy. The same reasons often explain why children
may get constipated on holiday. Incidentally, it is a good idea to
try and make sure that when children start school they get up
early enough to spend time in the lavatory without being hurried.

You'll have undoubtedly noticed that I haven't yet suggested
any laxatives that might be worth trying. I do not believe that
laxatives are ever the real answer. When constipation occurs in a
child it is either the result of a dietary problem, a psychological
problem or, quite rarely, some underlying physical abnormality.
Constipation is frequently made much worse and turned from a
minor problem into a major one by the continued use of powerful
laxatives.

When do we need to see a doctor?

If the simple remedies I've outlined don't work or if the
constipation is accompanied by pain or any other worrying

symptom then you should seek a doctor's advice straight away.

By itself constipation is not a health hazard but it can, quite rarely, be a sign of an underlying disorder which requires professional treatment. It is, however, really very uncommon for a baby's constipation to be caused by anything more than a dietary imbalance.

It is also important to remember that the straining that may accompany severe constipation can produce a split or fissure around the anus. The pain from such a lesion can itself cause an unwillingness to open the bowels.

Convulsions

What are they?
A convulsion is officially defined as an involuntary spasm or contraction of muscles. There may be one single spasm or the movement may be repeated several times. A fit is the same thing as a convulsion. The two words are really interchangeable.

What causes them?
The human brain is filled with millions of electrical connections and messages travel around the nervous system with the aid of electrical impulses. The human brain uses electricity, for example, to contract the muscles.

If for any reason there is an abnormal burst of electrical activity within the brain then all the pathways which were up until that moment filled with normal message-carrying impulses will be overwhelmed. As a result muscles all over the body will be stimulated to act in no logical sequence. The muscles of the legs may twitch, the arms may fly all over the place and the eyelid muscles flutter. Breathing may stop temporarily too and the muscles which control the bowels and the bladder may be affected. That's a convulsion and the unusual muscle activity is just a sign that there has been some sort of electrical storm inside the brain. The child isn't aware of what is going on by the way. He suffers no pain and won't remember anything about it afterwards. Indeed, he'll probably fall asleep.

The electrical storms that cause all this chaos can be produced in many ways. A low blood sugar can produce a fit. A thwarted child having a breath holding attack can have a convulsion. The commonest cause is a high temperature. It is pretty safe to say that when a child between six months and 5 years old has a fit *and* a high temperature then the two are probably linked.

What about epilepsy?
The word epilepsy is used to refer to fits which recur, often without there being any obvious explanation. Most children who have convulsions have one only. Epilepsy is discussed on page 127.

How do we make the diagnosis?
If your child has a high temperature and is aged between six months and 5 years then his convulsion is probably a febrile convulsion. If he loses consciousness and does not have a high temperature then some form of epilepsy may be a possible diagnosis. (See page 133 for how to use a thermometer.)

You should not, however, try to make a diagnosis yourself. You should follow the instructions given in the following paragraph and call your doctor so that he can make the diagnosis, initiate any tests he considers appropriate and offer the most suitable form of treatment.

What can we do?
1 Try not to panic. Between 5 and 10 per cent of all children will have convulsions at some time. Most of these will be febrile convulsions. The great majority of these convulsions will do no lasting harm.
2 Lie your child on his right side either on a bed or on the floor. Turn his face towards the floor so that if he vomits he will not choke or inhale any vomited material. (See page 72 for details about choking.)
3 Don't try to push a spoon or anything else between his teeth or gums.
4 Make sure your child doesn't do himself any damage by banging himself against any hard objects. Move furniture and so on out of the way.
5 If he has a high temperature try to cool him a little. Remove any clothing that you can remove easily. Open a window or turn on a fan if the temperature in the room is high. Use a sponge or cloth soaked in tepid water to wipe him down.
6 Telephone your doctor to let him know what is happening.

Most convulsions will last less than five minutes and so there is little chance of his being able to arrive before the convulsions are over.

7 Don't try giving anything to eat or drink either during or immediately after a convulsion. And don't try giving any medicines either unless your child has had previous convulsions and your doctor has given you specific drugs and specific instructions. You don't need to give artificial respiration to a child having a convulsion. And it isn't a good idea to put him in a bath of water. Children are more likely to be harmed by inappropriate treatment than by convulsions.

Are convulsions inherited?

If there is a family history of febrile convulsions then there is an increased risk of your child having a convulsion.

Do fits cause brain damage?

Convulsions in children are usually harmless – frightening but harmless. In one recent study of over 1700 children there were no cases of any lasting damage as a result of fits. There is certainly no truth in the suggestion that convulsions can cause permanent brain damage. Nor, incidentally, is there any truth in the suggestion that children who have convulsions will be more likely to develop epilepsy later on.

If our child has one convulsion is he more likely to have another?

Yes. If a child has one febrile convulsion then he is more likely to have another. But children are less likely to have febrile convulsions as they grow older. After the age of 3 the likelihood of your child having a febrile convulsion falls each year.

How can we stop our child having another febrile convulsion?

Any infection that affects your child can theoretically produce a convulsion if it also produces a high temperature. An ear infection, a throat infection or an attack of cystitis can all produce a high enough temperature to cause a convulsion. So can infectious diseases such as measles. It is the speed with which the temperature rises that seems to be more important than the final temperature that is achieved. A sudden rise of a few degrees is more likely to cause a convulsion than a slow, steady rise to an even higher temperature.

To prevent a febrile convulsion keep an eye on your child's temperature and his general condition. If his condition seems to be deteriorating and his temperature is rising then slow down the rate at which the temperature rises.

Remove as many of his clothes as you can, open the window if necessary and turn off the heating in his room. Tepid sponging is an excellent way to slow down the rate at which a temperature rises. Just dip a sponge or cloth in a bowl of lukewarm water and wipe it over your child's skin. Don't use cold water because that can have an effect opposite to that required. The cold water simply confuses the body's temperature control mechanism with the result that the body's own defences are organised in such a way so as to preserve as much heat as possible. Ice water and cold baths should be avoided for the same reason.

At the early stages of your child's illness there is some point in giving the appropriate dose of aspirin since this can help keep the temperature down. You should not give any other medicine or drugs unless these have been prescribed by your doctor and recommended specifically for this sort of situation. Give your child lots of fluids to drink.

When do we need to see the doctor?
Most febrile convulsions and indeed most other convulsions will be over long before the doctor can get to you or your child. But you should, nevertheless, call him and ask for advice. Only your doctor can really make a firm diagnosis as to the cause of the convulsion.

If your child's convulsion lasts for more than five or ten minutes and the doctor isn't actually on his way to you then you should take your child to the nearest hospital which has a casualty department.

What will the doctor do?
First of all he will want to be sure of the diagnosis. To do this he may need to arrange for your child to be admitted to hospital where tests can be done. There doctors may arrange for a lumbar puncture, X-rays, an electroencephalogram and blood tests.

Even if the diagnosis is certain there will probably be a need for some form of treatment. Unless the temperature has fallen fairly dramatically and any underlying infection has cleared up by itself your doctor will probably want to start your child on a course of antibiotics.

If there seems to be an enhanced risk that your child may suffer from a further convulsion the doctor may well decide to prescribe an anti-convulsant. This drug may need to be taken regularly or it may be provided simply for use in any future emergencies. Make sure you understand exactly how and when any anti-convulsant drug is to be used.

Coughing

What is it?

The human body contains an enormous number of marvellous automatic defence mechanisms designed to protect the internal workings of the human organism. One of these defence mechanisms is the cough reflex. If anything threatens to block the tubes leading down into the lungs a series of automatic responses are brought into action. These exist to thwart the threatened blockage. The cough reflex can prove life-saving. For example, the child who has a badly infected chest will be able to cough up material which might otherwise lie around in the lungs and make things worse. One of the problems doctors have to deal with when they are looking after patients who are deeply unconscious is that the cough reflex is absent. Without this vital reflex it is all too easy for phlegm and mucus to collect in the lungs and for infections such as pneumonia to develop.

What causes it?

The most dramatic type of cough is the one that is produced when some foreign object gets into the tubes leading down into the lungs. If a child who is otherwise quite well suddenly develops a cough then he may have inhaled a small object which is threatening to block part of a lung. This can happen when small children are playing with tiny objects. It is particularly likely to occur when children throw small sweets or peanuts up into the air and try catching them in their mouths.

The cough that frightens mothers most is probably the characteristic 'whoop' that gives whooping cough its name. This infection usually starts with the symptoms of an ordinary cold.

Then the child starts coughing and breathing in air through a partially closed trachea. It is the air going through this narrowed windpipe that produces the 'whoop'. Vomiting is very common with whooping cough since small children are often unable to spit out phlegm. They bring the phlegm up far enough to swallow it and the accumulation of phlegm in the stomach then makes them vomit.

Although coughing can be an important protective reflex it can also be quite unnecessary and very exhausting. The unnecessary cough that causes most distress is probably the one that lasts most of the night and keeps not only the sufferer awake but also his parents and possibly even the neighbours.

Night-time coughs are sometimes produced by mucus tickling down the back of the throat. This is particularly common when the child has a cold or is suffering from catarrh. Night-time coughs can also be produced if the temperature in the bedroom is different to the temperature in the rest of the house.

The other cause of a ticklish, unproductive cough that keeps everyone awake is cigarette smoke. The child who is breathing air heavy with cigarette smoke is very likely to acquire a persistent cough as he breathes in the polluted air.

Habit is the other extremely common cause of coughing. This type of cough, which is something of a nervous tic, is often a leftover from a cold or chest infection and it can be most aggravating for everyone.

What can we do about it?
The correct remedy for a cough depends upon the cause. The cough produced when a child has swallowed some foreign object doesn't need any treatment if the cough reflex does its job properly and the object is expelled. If the cough persists then you really ought to get medical attention straight away. If the child starts to choke as well as cough then you must try a first aid technique (see page 72).

If your child has a night-time cough that might be produced by mucus trickling down the back of his throat try giving him an extra pillow or encouraging him to try and sleep on his stomach instead of on his back.

If your child's cough might be caused by the fact that the temperature in his bedroom is lower than the temperature elsewhere in the house try putting a heater on in the bedroom for an hour or so before bedtime. Just taking the chill off is enough. Do be careful not to get the room too hot and stuffy for that too can trigger off a night-time cough!

The hot lemon drink described on page 81 can also be used to help alleviate a persistent cough. Most of the cough sweets and cough medicines that you can buy over the counter are useless since manufacturers are not allowed to include powerful drugs in any useful quantity.

When do we need to see the doctor?

If a child coughs up blood or is breathless then you should see the doctor without any delay. If coughing produces phlegm or is accompanied by vomiting then you should see the doctor. If there is any wheezing, rattling or whooping then you should see the doctor.

You should see the doctor about any cough that persists for more than five days.

Cradle cap

What is it?

Cradle cap consists of accumulated skin oil and dead cells which stick to the scalp in yellowish, scaly, crusted patches.

What causes it?

The sebaceous glands in the skin regularly produce a substance called sebum which helps to keep the skin oiled and healthy. And dead cells are always being pushed off the surface of the skin and replaced by fresh ones from beneath.

Under normal circumstances this mixture of dead cells and oil is removed from the skin and the scalp when we wash. However, babies have to be washed by their mothers and most mothers are rather afraid of rubbing too hard on the top of the head because of the so-called soft spots or fontanelle. That is the most common reason why babies get cradle cap.

How do we make the diagnosis?

The definition of cradle cap should make it fairly easy to diagnose accurately.

What can we do about it
If you carefully rub the part of the scalp on which the cradle cap has accumulated with a rough facecloth on which you've put a little soap then the problem will usually disappear. If the crust seems too hard for this simple treatment try rubbing a little olive oil into the scalp twelve hours before your baby's next bath.

If the cradle cap still persists then you can try a special shampoo. I suggest that you look for a shampoo containing coal tar, or salicylic acid. Make sure that none of the medicated shampoo gets into your child's eyes.

Do children with cradle cap always get eczema?
Children with cradle cap sometimes have similar patches on other parts of their skin but I don't know of any evidence that they are more likely to suffer from eczema, psoriasis or any other chronic skin problems.

These patches of dead cells and oil can usually be removed from the other parts of the body in much the same way that they can be removed from the scalp.

What do we need to see the doctor?
If you are certain about the diagnosis then you should be able to deal with the problem yourself. If you are not certain about the diagnosis or you fail to remove the patch of oil and cells then ask your doctor to help. He will probably prescribe a similar treatment if he agrees with your diagnosis.

Cramp

What is it?
A sudden, painful contraction of a muscle.

What causes it?
Sudden chilling can produce cramp pains or make cramp worse. Losing salt and body fluids also helps to produce cramp pains which are therefore common among athletes in the warmer months.

What can we do about it?
Cramp pains are produced by muscles being constricted and so

the pains can be relieved by relaxing the affected muscles. This is best done by forcibly contracting the opposing set of muscles.

So, for example, if it is the calf muscles which are contracted and painful the problem can be relieved by forcibly contracting the muscles at the front of the shin. This is done most readily by simply pushing the toes up in the direction of the knee.

Cramp pains in other muscles can be relieved in a similar way.

It is important to be aware of the risk of cramps developing when children are swimming. The risk is greater the colder the water and the major hazard is, of course, that the child will be unable to swim, will panic and may drown.

Can we prevent cramps developing?

If a child gets lots of night cramps it may be because the bedclothes are too heavy and are pulling the feet into a downward position. A bed cradle may help to keep the bedclothes off the feet. Failing that it may be enough to ensure that the bedclothes are tucked in less tightly. Alternatively a pillow placed at the bottom of the bed may physically prevent the feet from getting into a position where cramp will develop.

Regular cramp sufferers should try a simple exercise which often helps night cramps developing. The child simply removes his shoes and stands barefoot two or three feet away from a wall. Then, keeping his heels in contact with the floor, he leans forward so that his hands rest on the wall. He stays like this for ten seconds, rests for five seconds, and then repeats the exercise two or three times.

The child who does this every night for a fortnight should find that night cramps become a thing of the past.

Children who do a lot of sport and who get cramps should be given salt tablets according to the manufacturer's instructions.

Crying

What is it?

The first few times a newborn baby cries helps fill his lungs with air. There don't seem to be many other physiological benefits associated with crying – it is simply a non-specific reaction to physical, mental and emotional stress. For young babies in particular crying is the only reliable means of communication. It is used to denote boredom, hunger, tiredness, unhappiness, frustration and all other unpleasant experiences.

Tears are produced by the tear glands and are intended to help keep the eyes clear by washing away dust and dirt. No one really knows why crying should be accompanied by tears.

What causes it?

There are hundreds of reasons why a child should start crying. Here are some of the commonest problems.

1 Hunger As soon as children can talk they'll tell you when they're hungry. Small babies can't tell you what they want. And so they'll cry. A baby who hasn't had enough milk at one feed will often wake and start crying an hour later.

2 Pain All of us cry when we're in pain. The sounds we make are apparently quite different to the sounds we make when we cry in anger, frustration or misery. Researchers have shown that parents are often instantly able to identify a child's cry of pain and to differentiate between that and any other sort of crying. A child in acute or severe pain will often cry much louder than at any other time.

3 Loneliness Babies who are bored will often cry for extra attention. If they feel that they have been ignored or disregarded for long enough then they'll start crying. For the first few months of life babies need all the comfort and love they can get.

4 Teething Babies are sometimes irritable and likely to cry when they're teething (see page 229).

5 Colic Three month colic usually occurs at the busiest time of day for most mothers – the early evening when husband has just come home and wants his dinner and the other children are being prepared for bed. The crying of three month colic may be produced by the baby's awareness of the stress existing in the household. Three month colic is, therefore, one of the earliest stress diseases (see page 79).

6 Discomfort The baby who is in a draught, who has wind or who is too hot, too cold or too wet will cry to draw attention to his problem. Crying is all he can do to get his problem solved.

7 Illness Crying is often an early non-specific symptom of illness. If your baby or child cries persistently or particularly loudly and you can't find a cause then you should consider the possibility that he is either sickening for something or already has something!

8 Sadness and depression Children can get depressed, miserable or just plain sad just as adults can. It is quite normal for a child to cry occasionally because he is sad but if the crying is accompanied by apathy or aggression then a more serious depression may be the problem.

How do we make the diagnosis?

With time most parents become very good at knowing why their child is crying. If you don't know why he is crying, if you don't seem able to stop him crying, if the crying is in any way unusual or if the crying is particularly persistent then you should ask for your doctor's advice. There isn't usually any reason why you shouldn't wrap your baby up and take him along to the doctor's clinic rather than wait for a home visit. Medical advice should also be sought if the crying is accompanied by any other symptoms which suggest illness. If, for example, your child looks unusual, behaves oddly, won't eat, vomits, has a high temperature or is particularly sleepy then you need professional help.

Cuts

What can we do about them?

If the cut is very small you won't need to do anything about it. The body's own defence mechanisms will prove entirely adequate and will both cleanse and heal the wound. If you want to do something to a cut that is less than half an inch long I suggest that you confine yourself to washing the wound with plenty of fresh running water and perhaps a little liquid antiseptic. If the wound gapes and doesn't seem likely to heal because the edges are too far apart then a piece of sticking plaster left in position for no more than twenty-four hours will help. You can buy small 'butterfly sutures' from pharmacies and although these are rather expensive they are extremely useful for helping small wounds heal without scars.

I don't recommend that you use antiseptic creams, waterproof sticking plasters or any of the proprietary medicines recommended for cuts and grazes. Antiseptic creams make the wounds sticky and impede rather than assist healing. Waterproof plasters seal off the wound and make infection more likely.

If your child is not protected against tetanus or has not had a booster injection within the last twelve months then a tetanus injection is required however small the wound may be. Tetanus spores can get into the body through pricks let alone small cuts.

When do we need to see the doctor?
You may need to see the doctor if the cut is more than an inch long, if your child suffers from any blood disorder which makes it likely that the normal clotting mechanism will not work or if the bleeding does not stop within twenty minutes. If the cut is less than an inch long, is purely superficial, is clean and does not gape then you can probably leave the body's own defence mechanisms to cope with the problem.

Cystitis

What is it?
The word cystitis literally means an inflammation of the bladder.

What causes it?
Cystitis is usually caused by an infection of the urinary tract. It is much commoner in girls than in boys because the urethra (which connects the bladder to the outside world) is much shorter in girls than in boys. The bacteria can travel up the relatively short female urethra much quicker and easier than they can travel up the longer male urethra.

If there is any abnormality of the urinary tract then the chances of a child developing cystitis are greater.

How do we make the diagnosis?
The symptoms of cystitis are: a desire to pass urine more often than usual, a need to go immediately, a stinging pain on passing urine and a feeling that the bladder still needs emptying even

though it is quite apparent that there isn't anything left to be passed!

These symptoms are fairly obvious in older children but in younger children the disease is extremely difficult to detect because the symptoms themselves are not always recognised. Because of this difficulty in recognising the symptoms doctors will usually test the urine routinely when young children seem miserable and no explanation can be found.

What can we do about it?

A hot-water bottle will relieve any accompanying abdominal pain. It helps to give your child frequent drinks since the more fluid is taken the quicker the infection will be washed out of the system.

Apart from these simple measures there isn't any other remedy that I recommend for children with cystitis. If the symptoms suggest this diagnosis then a doctor's advice should be sought.

When should we see the doctor?

Whenever the symptoms suggest a diagnosis of cystitis.

What will the doctor do?

He'll probably begin by asking you to provide him with a urine sample for the laboratory to use for some simple tests. This urine sample needs to be collected in a sterile container (so that it is not contaminated by bacteria that are already present in the container) and it needs to be a mid-stream specimen. (This means that the sample shouldn't be the first part of the stream but should be taken once the stream has become established. This ensures that the sample is not contaminated by any bacteria that happened to be on the skin outside the urethra.)

Urine samples for this type of test do not have to be early morning specimens. It is only for pregnancy tests that urine samples need to be taken first thing in the morning.

The laboratory will attempt to grow any bacteria that happen to be in the urine and they will then do special tests to find out which antibiotics those bacteria are susceptible to. Once they have completed these investigations they will be able to advise your doctor of the most suitable drug to use.

If cystitis persists or recurs then additional investigations will probably be necessary. These may involve special X-rays of the urinary tract, including the bladder and the kidneys.

How can we prevent cystitis?

There isn't much that can be done for boys to prevent infections getting into the bladder but to help girls stop the spread of infection ensure that the bottom is wiped from front to back. This ensures the bacteria in and round the anus are wiped away from the urethra and not towards it.

Deafness

What types of deafness are there?

Children can be permanently deaf, temporarily deaf, partly deaf or completely deaf. Children who are permanently and completely deaf need most help but other children will also need a considerable amount of support and understanding.

Children can be born deaf or they can become deaf after birth.

What causes deafness?

In the normal healthy ear sound waves pass down the ear canal to the drum. There the sound waves make the drum vibrate; those vibrations are in turn transmitted across the middle ear by the three bones known as the malleus, the incus and the stapes. From the middle ear the vibrations are passed on to the inner ear. This contains a special organ called the cochlea which converts the vibrations into electrical impulses. These impulses are then carried via a special nerve to the brain. (The inner ear also contains the semicircular canals which control the sense of balance.)

Any damage, disease or malfunction which affects one or both ears or which affects the external canal, the bones of the middle ear, the inner ear or the nerve which carries impulses to the brain can cause deafness. The extent and site of the damage will decide the extent of the deafness.

The external canal can be quite easily blocked by wax, small beads, bits of food or by inflammation and infection. The blockage, whatever causes it, will stop sound waves passing down to the drum. Deafness produced by a temporary blockage of the canal is relatively easy to deal with.

The drum itself and the bones which carry the sound waves

across the middle ear to the inner ear are most commonly damaged by infection. The name otitis media is given to the special type of infection which affects this part of the ear specifically. The type of deafness produced by otitis media is usually temporary but occasionally the damage can be so severe that there is some permanent hearing loss. Unless the ear infection spreads to both sides the hearing loss will usually only affect one ear.

Injury, infection and congenital malformations can all cause the inner ear organ to work ineffectively and can all be responsible for a failure of the nerve which carries sounds to the brain. When a child is born completely deaf the chances are fairly high that the deafness is caused by a fault in the nerve.

How can we tell that our child is deaf?

With small babies up to three months of age the only way to test for deafness is to look for some response to loud noises or voices with which the baby might have been expected to become familiar. If there is no response at all then deafness must be suspected although the diagnosis is by no means certain at this stage.

Babies between three and twelve months of age should not only notice sounds but they should be turning their heads towards the sounds they hear and beginning to make noises of their own. As they approach their first birthday most babies will be able to identify the source of any sound they hear and if they hear it repeatedly coming from the same place they will have learnt how to ignore it. This last point is important because the deaf child who is approaching his first birthday may be just beginning to respond to loud noises.

Some time between their first and second birthdays most children start talking. By the time they have reached their second birthdays most children will be able to construct very short sentences. Deafness should be suspected if these milestones aren't reached. The deaf child can't learn to talk because he can't hear other people speaking.

In older children partial deafness can be detected if a child fails to learn how to speak so that strangers can understand him or if he has learning problems at school. By the age of 5 or 6 most children will be able to speak fairly clearly and should be picking up new information at school at quite a rapid rate.

Why are deaf children also mute?

Children learn to speak entirely by imitating what they hear. The deaf child can't hear and so he can't imitate.

It is important that deafness be detected at an early stage so that the child can be given whatever aids are likely to be useful as soon as possible. The deaf child who can be provided with a hearing aid may then be able to learn how to speak.

Can deafness be prevented?

Some forms of congenital deafness can't be prevented but one of the commonest forms of deafness is that produced by german measles infection. This can be prevented. All women who are planning to become pregnant should ensure that they are protected against german measles.

One of the most important causes of deafness in children is infection of the middle ear. This particular type of problem can usually be prevented if ear infections are dealt with swiftly and effectively. Ordinary ear infections do not usually cause deafness and problems usually only become really apparent when infections are allowed to persist.

One other possible cause of deafness should also be borne in mind. It has been known for some time that repeated exposure to loud noises can cause deafness and it is an established fact that exposure to loud music in particular can cause permanent damage. Many quite young children enjoy loud music and now play music with the aid of stereo headphones. Children should be warned of the hazards which can be associated with loud music.

Finally, it is important to remember to resist the temptation to poke anything smaller than your foot into a child's ear. It is very easy to damage the drum and the middle ear by the unskilled use of needles, cotton wool swabs and so on.

What can we do about it?

If you suspect that there is something wrong with your child's hearing then you should ask your doctor to arrange for hearing tests as soon as possible. Temporary partial hearing loss with head colds, catarrh and stuffiness is common. Anything more complete or more lasting merits professional attention.

If your child is found to be deaf then there are many ways in which you can help.

The most important single thing you can do is to talk to your child just as much as you possibly can. Talk so that he can see you talking and try to keep your hands and head still so that he can concentrate on watching your face. Don't be tempted to shout, don't talk very slowly, don't exaggerate lip movements and don't talk in that strange way that so many people adopt when they're talking to folk who are hard of hearing.

It will help if you can find the time and the patience to explain things and to let your child see the actions which match the words you are using. Try and ensure that your child becomes independent, that he is subject to discipline, that he isn't left out of any conversations and that he wears any hearing aid that has been supplied.

Don't talk to him from another room because he won't be able to see your face. Do try not to mumble. Rephrase your words and try to include longer words if he doesn't understand you. Longer words are easier to lip read. Don't cover your mouth when you talk. And do call his name before you speak to him to make sure that he is paying full attention.

When should we see the doctor?
You should seek medical advice as soon as you suspect that there might be some hearing loss. Even quite mild hearing loss can produce a fairly severe speech impediment if your child is not able to differentiate properly between different sounds.

What will the doctor do?
Your doctor will probably begin by doing some simple tests designed to gauge the approximate extent of any deafness. If, as a result of these simple tests, he suspects that there is any loss of hearing acuity he will then arrange for more formal tests to be done. The instrument used to measure hearing is called an audiometer. It produces different sounds at different levels and the technician operating the machine will be able to plot a graph which shows just where the child's hearing acuity is strongest and where any weak points lie.

Once these tests have been done a firm diagnosis as to the cause and site will need to be made. The doctor's initial examination will have ruled out such causes as wax in the external canal. The task now will be to decide whether the hearing loss is due to damage in the middle ear, in the inner ear or in the nerve which carries impulses to the brain.

If an operation can be done to help relieve the hearing loss this will be arranged. In many cases, however, there will not be any such simple solution and a hearing aid will have to be provided. It is important that both parents and child know how to use such an aid and are fully aware of its capabilities and its limitations.

Hearing aids

Hearing aids don't provide normal hearing and don't have any curative effect on the ear. Nor will they help someone who is completely deaf. All they do is amplify normal sounds so that they can be heard more readily. Modern hearing aids are much more effective and far less cumbersome than the old-fashioned speaking trumpets that the deaf had to use just a few years ago. The availability of miniature batteries has made it possible to produce tiny aids.

If your child needs a hearing aid you should listen to your doctor's advice. There are many commercial organisations selling hearing aids but I don't recommend that you visit any of them without having first asked for professional medical advice. The people selling hearing aids have a vested interest in selling you a particular type of aid. The doctor you see should have no commercial interests at all. He should only be concerned to ensure that your child is fitted with the most suitable aid available.

In addition to your own doctor you will almost certainly be able to talk to specialists who can describe to you the ways in which the recommended aid should be worn and used.

Other aids

In addition to aids designed to amplify sounds there are a number of other aids available for deaf people. It is, for example, possible to arrange for doorbells to be connected to house lights and it is possible to obtain alarm clocks which operate flashing lights instead of ringing bells.

What about sign language?

Deaf people who cannot lip read often use sign language to communicate with others. There are some finger and hand signs which stand for whole words and some movements and positions which spell out separate letters.

Sadly sign language is not universal and there are, for example,

some differences in the signs used by English-speaking people
and French-speaking people.

Diabetes

What is it?

Under normal circumstances the pancreas gland produces a
substance called insulin used by the body in the breakdown of
sugar. When the production of insulin is for any reason impaired
the body's capacity to deal effectively with sugar is reduced.
Diabetes mellitus, or sugar diabetes, is the name given to the
condition in which the pancreas fails to produce the amount of
insulin the body needs.

When diabetes develops in adults it is often fairly mild and the
condition can then be dealt with either by limiting the amount of
sugar in the diet or by using drugs which stimulate the pancreas
to produce more insulin. When diabetes develops in children,
however, the condition tends to be more serious. It is usually
necessary to reduce the intake of sugar and to give insulin by
injection. Insulin cannot be given by mouth because it is de-
activated in the stomach. The amounts of sugar and insulin given
need to be adjusted carefully so that the two are balanced
precisely. Under normal circumstances the healthy pancreas
balances its own production of insulin to match the amount of
sugar which needs metabolising. In the diabetic child this
equation has to be managed by those with the responsibility for
controlling the diet and insulin intake.

What causes it?

The disease is caused by a failure of the pancreas gland to
produce insulin. It is usually a genetically transmitted disease and
although a child's parents may not have the disease there is
usually a family history of diabetes.

When can it develop?

Diabetes can develop at any age. Generally speaking the later
the onset the less serious the problem will be.

How common is it?

About 2 per cent of the population are said to have diabetes but only about one in twenty of those are children. The rest are adults of various ages.

How do we make the diagnosis?

The earliest signs of developing diabetes are usually an excessive thirst, a tendency to pass a good deal of urine and an exceptional hunger. Tiredness, irritability and weight loss may also occur. Bedwetting is sometimes an early indication of diabetes. It is impossible to make a complete diagnosis without a urine test or blood test but if any of the symptoms listed here occur then medical advice should be sought.

If there is any family history of diabetes then this fact should be made known to the family doctor as soon as possible after the child's birth so that this fact can be recorded on the medical notes.

What can we do about it?

You should learn as much as you can about your child's condition and about diabetes in general. Diabetes cannot be cured but it is not usually a difficult disease to control and when the condition is controlled effectively complications will be relatively rare.

When should we see the doctor?

You should see the doctor as soon as possible if you suspect that your child might have diabetes. And you should seek his advice at once if you are unhappy about the condition of any child known to have diabetes.

When do insulin injections have to be given?

This depends on the nature of the diabetes and the type of insulin being used. Some forms of insulin act rapidly while others have an effect within the body for a much longer period of time. The dose of insulin and the time it has to be given will be decided by the child's own doctor and possibly by a paediatrician or a specialist in diabetes. Insulin injections usually need to be given at least once a day.

Who gives the insulin injections?

It doesn't really matter who gives the injections but it is obviously less convenient for everyone concerned if the injections have to be given by a nurse. Generally speaking it is best for the patient to give his or her own injections. Children from the age of 4 can usually manage to do this quite safely and effectively. It is important to tell children as much as possible about their condition so that they understand exactly what they can and cannot do.

Will our doctor arrange an appointment at the hospital?
Most general practitioners refer their young diabetic patients to a local specialist for advice but from then on they will usually share the care. Young diabetics often need to go into hospital to begin with to have their diabetes stabilised.

What complications are there?
The two common problems which affect diabetics occur when there is too much insulin given and when there is too little insulin given. If the amount of insulin in the body is too great then the amount of sugar available will fall too low. This condition is known as hypoglycaemia. If there is too little insulin the amount of sugar will rise too high. This condition is known as hyperglycaemia.

It is often difficult to differentiate between the two basic extremes since in both cases the child will usually be drifting into unconsciousness. Generally speaking, however, it is usually considered safest to regard any weakness or faintness as having been produced by hypoglycaemia and to give a sweet drink or lump of sugar as an emergency measure. It is for this reason that diabetics are encouraged to carry with them sugar lumps or sweets. If a diabetic child loses consciousness it is vitally important to obtain medical help without any delay. Don't try giving sugar to an unconscious child. If a child has a hypoglycaemic attack but recovers after taking extra sugar then medical advice should be sought as soon as is convenient since it may be necessary to adjust the regular insulin dose.

Early signs of poor control include pallor, sweating, trembling and yawning. Children whose diabetes is out of control may also stagger when they walk around and they may be unusually irritable. For all these symptoms it is best to give a couple of lumps of sugar.

The other important complications associated with diabetes are usually the result of the blood sugar remaining too high for long periods of time. When this happens all the organs and tissues of the body can be adversely affected since the sugar rich blood may impair the circulation. If a diabetic child is managed carefully and successfully the risk of complications of this kind ensuing can be minimised.

What about diet?

It is as important to regulate the intake of food as it is to regulate the intake of insulin. Balancing food to insulin and vice versa is usually done automatically within the tissues but when the amount of insulin available is regulated artificially then the amount of food available must also be artificially regulated within fairly strict limits. Most diabetic specialists work with dieticians who will explain at length precisely how the diet should be controlled.

There are today some specialists who believe that diabetes is best controlled by adjusting the level of insulin to cope with the child's normal dietary intake. They argue that controlling the diet within rigid limits puts too much of a strain on the child and may limit his growth. You should follow your own physician's advice and stick to it.

How do we regulate the diet and the insulin? How do we know in advance if everything is all right?

You'll be given and shown how to use simple equipment with which you will be able to test your child's urine. This will tell you just how much sugar is present in the urine and, therefore, whether the insulin level needs to be increased or reduced. With a little practice and experience you'll be able to adjust the intake of insulin to cope with special parties and so on. It is also important to remember that when a child is taking more exercise than usual he will burn up sugar at a faster rate and so he will need less insulin.

What happens when the diabetic child is ill with something else?

As a general rule the amount of insulin given should be increased when there is an infection and increased if the child is taking considerably less exercise than usual. The size of the increase is best adjusted after testing the urine. When a child is ill this should be done two to four times a day with either the special tablets or strips provided.

Diarrhoea

What is it?

It is easier and safer to diagnose diarrhoea on the consistency of
the stool than on the frequency with which stools are passed.
When stools or motions are liquid or semi-liquid then a diagnosis
of diarrhoea should be made. If liquid stools are passed
frequently then the condition is probably bad diarrhoea. If, on the
other hand, stools are passed frequently but are firm and well
formed then a diagnosis of diarrhoea should not be made.

What causes it

In babies and small children diarrhoea is a common consequence of a feeding problem. If there is too much fat in the
baby's feed then the stools will be soft, greasy and rather yellow.
If the feed contains too much carbohydrate the stools will be soft,
yellow and rather frothy. Breast fed babies sometimes have very
loose, rather sparse greenish stools as do babies who aren't
getting enough to eat. Too much sugar in the feed can cause
diarrhoea and in children who are recovering from gastroenteritis milk itself can cause diarrhoea since the bowel can be
damaged in such a way that the digestion of the substances in
milk is affected. In older children too much fruit is a common
cause of diarrhoea. In all these cases the baby will look quite
well and will not have any other obvious signs or symptoms of
illness.

Infections are, of course, an extremely common cause of
diarrhoea in children. Gastroenteritis is a possible diagnosis
when the diarrhoea is accompanied by vomiting and this
condition needs to be taken very seriously. Less serious attacks
of diarrhoea can accompany just about all other types of infection
– including respiratory tract infections, for example.

Food poisoning is another cause of diarrhoea which usually
also causes some vomiting. Some types of food poisoning,
dysentery for example, are extremely infectious and will spread
around schools and homes very rapidly. Food allergies are fairly
common causes of diarrhoea (see page 138).

Antibiotics, appendicitis and anxiety are three additional
common causes of diarrhoea. Antibiotics produce diarrhoea by
interfering with the bacterial inhabitants of the intestinal tract,
appendicitis produces diarrhoea in some children but not in

others while anxiety is a well-established cause of diarrhoea in both children and adults.

Paradoxically children who are constipated may occasionally develop diarrhoea and incontinence as motions slowly seep round the blockage.

How do we make the diagnosis?

Deciding exactly what has caused diarrhoea is a difficult job and it is one that I think is largely irrelevant since the main question parents need to answer is not 'What has caused the diarrhoea?' but 'Is it serious?'.

Answering that question when the patient is a baby or an infant below the age of 1 year is rather different to answering it when the patient is an older child. Babies and infants are particularly likely to become dehydrated if they suffer from diarrhoea and this risk is intensified if the diarrhoea is accompanied by vomiting. With older children the risk of dehydration accompanying diarrhoea alone diminishes fairly rapidly as the child ages while the risk of dehydration accompanying diarrhoea and vomiting diminishes at a slightly slower rate.

To diagnose dehydration it is usually suggested that parents study their child's skin, since the dehydrated child will have less elastic skin than usual. To test for elasticity all you do is pick up a pinch of skin. In the normal child the skin will immediately move back into its normal position when you release your hold. In the dehydrated child the skin will remain in a slightly pinched position for a few seconds.

Although this test for dehydration is very useful in most children it is of less value in children who are overweight. The excess fat means that there will be very few obvious changes in the consistency of the skin. In these circumstances it is important to look for other signs as well. I suggest that parents be on the watch for sunken eyes, a dry mouth and rapid breathing.

Those are the serious signs, however, and most cases of diarrhoea should be dealt with effectively well before that stage is reached.

What can we do about it?

When diarrhoea is caused by a feeding problem the remedy won't be too difficult to find. A change in the type of formula or the constitution of the mix for bottle fed babies may provide an adequate answer, for example.

If the diarrhoea is caused by anxiety then reassurance, time and comfort may be all that is needed.

If the diarrhoea is caused by an antibiotic given for some other problem then it may help to give daily yoghurt. This apparently bizarre solution works by helping the body to restock with its normal variety of inoffensive bacteria and thereby resist the attempts of potentially damaging bacteria to colonise the bowel. Apart from using yoghurt in these particular circumstances I don't really think that there is any point in using any medicines for the treatment of diarrhoea. The medicines that are mild enough to be safe are ineffective.

To help prevent diarrhoea causing dehydration bottle fed babies should be given extra feeds of water and breast fed babies should be given extra feeds on the breast. For bottle fed babies milk feeds should either be cut out or reduced in strength. It is usually wise to avoid solids altogether until the diarrhoea has settled.

When diarrhoea is accompanied by vomiting you should avoid giving anything at all by mouth apart from water. If a child who is vomiting and also has diarrhoea looks ill, has a fever, or shows any signs of dehydration then you should seek medical advice as soon as you possibly can. It is also important to seek advice if diarrhoea persists for more than a day or two. There are some conditions, such as coeliac disease and chronic ulcerative colitis, in which persistent diarrhoea (which may or may not be accompanied by the passage of mucus or blood) is an important early sign which suggests that treatment may be required.

Once the diarrhoea has begun to settle get your child back to a normal diet fairly gently. It will probably be two or three days before your child is able to cope with his normal diet again.

How can we prevent diarrhoea developing?

If anyone in your home has diarrhoea it is important to ensure that rules of hygiene are followed very strictly. If you travel abroad you should be particularly careful not to allow your child to drink unboiled water or milk or to eat foods or drinks made with unboiled milk or water or washed in unboiled water. Fuller instructions about staying healthy when travelling abroad appear on page 308.

When should we see the doctor?

You should see the doctor if your child with diarrhoea:

1 Seems ill or has a fever.
2 Passes any blood together with the diarrhoea.
3 Has recurring bouts of diarrhoea.
4 Shows any signs of dehydration.
5 Has accompanying vomiting that lasts for more than twenty-four hours.
6 Has diarrhoea for more than forty-eight hours.

What will the doctor do?

The doctor will, if he thinks it necessary, arrange for tests to be done to decide exactly what is causing the diarrhoea. These tests may include an examination of a sample of the child's faeces in the laboratory and an attempt to isolate any organism which might be causing the diarrhoea. If the diarrhoea has persisted for some time or is a recurring problem he may arrange for an internal examination of the bowel with a sigmoidoscope or he may arrange for special X-rays such as a barium enema examination.

Any fluid loss and accompanying dehydration will be repaired by carefully arranged feeding or by replacing lost fluid with the aid of an intravenous drip. Sometimes your doctor will arrange for your child to be admitted to hospital. This is often done not because the child is so seriously ill that hospital care is essential but because admission to hospital is the best way to ensure that no serious complications (such as dehydration) do develop.

Dyslexia

What is it?

The child who suffers from dyslexia finds it difficult to use words. He will be slow to learn to read, to learn to write and to learn how to spell properly.

Many parents wrongly assume that any child who is a little slower than average at learning to read must be dyslexic. This is not necessarily so since children learn to read and master words at different rates and it is far commoner for a child to be simply a little slow at learning to read than it is for him to be frankly dyslexic.

What causes it?
Dyslexia is a specific learning difficulty caused by a specific disorder within the brain.

How do we make the diagnosis?
1 The dyslexic child will usually be slower to learn how to use words than to use figures. He will usually show a very specific deficiency in this one area of learning alone. In oral classwork, mental arithmetic and so on the child will usually be as good as any other members of his form.
2 Dyslexic children often get confused by individual letters; frequently writing them down back to front or upside down.
3 There will often be a family history of a reading problem. Dyslexia is three times as common in boys as in girls.
4 Children who learn to speak rather late seem to have a higher incidence of dyslexia.
5 Children who are ambidextrous seem more likely to be dyslexic. This is because there is an absence of dominance between the two halves of the brain.
6 Dyslexia seems to be more common in children who are clumsy.
7 Dyslexia often produces other problems. The child who has difficulty with the written word may become withdrawn or aggressive as a result of problems at school. He may show physical signs of stress (see page 290).

How common is it?
Some experts believe that dyslexia is far commoner than is suspected. One estimate is that one in twenty-five children suffer from dyslexia.

When do we need the doctor?
If you think your child could be dyslexic then you should seek medical help straightaway.

What will the doctor do?
Your doctor will probably arrange a referral to an appropriate specialist. Speech therapists, psychologists and paediatricians

work together to help dyslexic children. Special lessons will usually be needed and you can help your child best by providing support and encouragement. The dyslexic child will have little confidence and will need a good deal of support from his parents.

Ear piercing

Is it safe?
Ear piercing is safe if it is done with sterile instruments. If it is done with dirty needles or with equipment which has not been properly cleaned there is a great risk of infection.

At what age is ear piercing safe?
Small children have a tendency to wriggle about. That makes ear piercing difficult and even dangerous. Infection is possible unless the child keeps the pierced ear site clean. Apart from that there are no other reasons why children shouldn't have their ears pierced at any age they and their parents favour.

Earache

What causes it?
A narrow tube connects the ear to the nose and if, as a result of a head cold, an infection of the glands or an allergy of any kind, this tube becomes blocked then the pressure change which result produce pain inside the ear. This pain can be persistent or intermittent, mild or excruciating and may or may not be accompanied by any other signs.

That is the commonest cause of earache but there are other causes. If there is any foreign object inside the ear, that can cause pain. Impacted wax can produce pain too, as can boils and localised infections.

Earache can also be produced by problems elsewhere in the head. Bad teeth, a sore throat and mumps can all cause earache. In addition earache can be produced by cold weather or cold winds – the cold produces muscle spasm and that causes the pain.

How do we make the diagnosis?

If earache occurs temporarily and briefly after a spell outside in the cold then it can be safely ignored. In any other circumstances earache needs to be investigated by a doctor. Only he has the training and equipment to look inside the ear and examine the state of the ear drums.

In very small children persistent crying for no obvious reason is often caused by earache. If a young child pulls on his ear or rubs his ear then that should be taken as a sign of earache.

What can we do about it?

While waiting for medical advice, relieve the pain of earache by filling a hot-water bottle, wrapping it in a thin towel or a pillow case and placing it against the ear. The warmth will usually relieve the pain very effectively. Painkillers such as aspirin or paracetamol are also useful.

I do not recommend that you use any of the proprietary drops or medicines designed to be put directly into the ear. Under some circumstances, when for example the ear drum is ruptured, these can produce complications of their own.

Is earache infectious?

No. In most circumstances, even if the earache is caused by an ear infection, the condition will not be infectious.

Does hair washing make earache worse?

No. As long as water doesn't flood the ear there is no reason why a child with earache shouldn't have a bath and have his hair washed.

Can swimming cause earache?

Yes. The ear's defences seem to be lowered by constant soaking in water. There doesn't seem to be any evidence to suggest that heavily chlorinated water is worse than unchlorinated water. Children with colds shouldn't go swimming since the combination of lowered defences and cold bugs will very possibly produce earache.

How can we tell whether the pain is inside the ear or in the outer ear?

If you really want to know where the infection is you can try tugging gently on the ear lobe. If the pain is produced by an infection deep inside the ear this won't make any difference. If the pain is produced by an infection in the outer ear this will cause additional pain. Either way a doctor's advice is required so the test is perhaps rather unnecessary.

What happens when there is a discharge from the ear?

When the eustachian tube (the tube which connects the ear to the throat and nose) is blocked it seals off the middle ear. Secretions continue to pour into this space but the secretions are now trapped. If and when these secretions become infected pus will form. This pus will put pressure on the eardrum and cause pain. Eventually the pressure may be great enough to rupture the ear drum. When that happens, pus, accompanied sometimes by blood, will flow from the outer ear. Because the ruptured drum is no longer under so much pressure the earache may be relieved as the fluid escapes.

A ruptured ear drum will usually heal without any difficulty and the child will be able to hear quite normally afterwards. Normally it is only when the ear drum is ruptured repeatedly that a hearing loss will be produced.

When do we need to see the doctor?

Whenever a child complains of an earache which is obviously not a temporary consequence of cold weather. It is important to have ear complaints treated as soon as possible in order to prevent recurrent damage to the drum. Most children who have a lot of ear trouble grow out of it when they reach the age of 8 or 9 and their ear drainage system becomes better developed and more effective.

What will the doctor do?

If the pain is caused by an obstruction the doctor will remove it. If it is caused by an infection then the doctor will probably treat the infection by prescribing an antibiotic. If the pain is severe and persistent and is caused by great pressure inside the ear an ear, nose and throat specialist may make a small hole in the eardrum to release the pus. Children who have recurrent ear infections sometimes have small plastic tubes inserted into their drums. These tubes allow pus to drain out without any pressure, any rupture of the drum or any consequent damage. These artificial tubes also allow air to get into that middle space and they assist drainage down the eustachian tube.

Ears that stick out

What causes it?

Some people have big noses. Others have small noses. Some people are tall. Others are short. Some people have neat, shell-like ears. Others have large ears that stick out a lot.

Does the shape of the ear have any effect on hearing?

No.

Does taping down the ears help to improve their appearance?

No.

What can be done?

A carefully designed hairstyle will hide ears that are considered unsightly. In really bad cases plastic surgery is a useful answer. Ask your own family doctor to arrange a referral to a plastic surgeon if you are contemplating the surgical alternative.

Eczema

What is it?

The two words 'eczema' and 'dermatitis' cause a great deal of confusion. There is really no need for any confusion for the two words are interchangeable. In this book I'm going to use the word 'eczema'.

Whatever terminology may be used the condition is fairly easy to diagnose. The skin is usually dry, reddened, itchy and swollen although weeping from blistered, raw-looking skin is also quite common. The fluid that has leaked may dry to form a crust. Because the affected area is usually itchy it may get scratched and thereby become infected.

Eczema occurs in about 10 per cent of all children although the severity obviously varies a good deal.

What causes it?

A vast number of very different problems may cause the symptoms of eczema.

1 Irritant eczema The skin can be irritated by a remarkably large range of substances. In babies and small children the commonest irritant is saliva which can reach the skin either through dribbling or through repeated licking of the skin around the lips. Nappy rash is another common variety of irritant eczema – in this case it is the ammonia in the urine-soaked nappy which produces the reaction in the skin.

Detergents, bleaches and soap powders are also common irritants.

2 Allergic contact eczema If a child becomes allergic to a particular substance then he will develop symptoms of eczema on contact with that substance. Individuals do not always become allergic to substances after one contact – sometimes an allergy only develops after repeated exposure over weeks, months or even years.

When an attack of eczema is caused by an allergy reaction to a particular substance the skin symptoms are similar to those which occur in irritant eczema. The most significant difference is that allergens can be identified by patch testing whereas irritants can only be identified by a process of elimination.

The commonest causes of allergic contact eczema in children are nickel, rubber, sticking plaster, some chemicals used in the manufacture of toys and a number of household plants.

3 Allergic eczema Skin rashes of the eczema type can be caused by eating certain types of food or by swallowing drugs to which an allergy response has been acquired. Penicillin and sulphonamide, two popularly prescribed anti-infective drugs, are perhaps the commonest pharmaceutical causes of allergic eczema. Almost any foods can cause allergy eczema but most problems are produced by eggs and dairy produce.

4 Inherited eczema The commonest type of eczema seen in small children is the inherited variety which is sometimes known as 'atopic eczema'. This usually develops between the ages of three months and 2 years of age and starts first on the face and nappy area, spreading in later years to the neck, hands, wrists and the fronts of the arms and legs. In many cases inherited eczema seems to diminish by the time a child reaches the age of 5 years.

There is firm evidence to show this type of eczema is less common in children who have been breast fed than in children who have been fed on cows' milk. Experts now believe that it is seven times as common in children who have been bottle fed as it is in children who have been fed with breast milk. The risks of developing eczema seem to vary directly in proportion to the total amount of milk consumed.

Mothers often wonder about the relationship between eczema and asthma. It is true that children who suffer from eczema may also suffer in later years from asthma or hay fever but the relationship is by no means inevitable.

It is in practice impossible to differentiate clearly between these different types of eczema. In some cases there may be a mixture of several types – with a child who has an inherited susceptibility to eczema suffering an allergy reaction to a specific allergen and then also suffering as a result of an irritant which has also been in contact with the skin. Mixed forms of eczema are extremely common.

The confusion is made even worse by the fact that a large number of very vague and often misleading terms are used by doctors when describing different types of eczema!

How do we make the diagnosis?
Try and decide what is causing your child's eczema. If you can identify a specific irritant or allergen then you may be able to deal with the eczema by avoiding the cause. Sadly, it isn't always possible to identify a specific cause when a child develops eczema. It is not even always possible to differentiate between irritant forms of eczema and allergic forms of eczema.

The table below is designed to help in making a diagnosis.

1 Eczema involving the entire body It is most likely to be due to an allergen that has been swallowed. Drugs are probably the most likely culprits. The skin sometimes takes ten days to respond to internal allergens.

2 Eczema confined to the area around the mouth Saliva is the most likely cause. You should also think of medicines, sweets, toothpaste and even lipsticks and other cosmetics.

3 Eczema confined to the ears Spectacle frames, earrings, ear studs and hearing aids can all produce eczema.

4 Eczema confined to the scalp Shampoo and other cosmetics are common causes of skin problems on the scalp.

5 Eczema confined to the area around the eyes and nose Cosmetics and skin creams must be considered as possible culprits. However, children will frequently touch their eyes and noses with other substances on their fingers. The eczema may or may not also involve the hands.

6 Eczema confined to the trunk The condition may have been caused by an irritant reaction or by an allergy reaction. If the response is of the allergic type then there will probably be a delay of some days between exposure to the allergen and the development of the skin reaction. This makes it even more difficult to form a firm diagnosis.

Clothes are a common cause of reactions. Buckles, belts, press-studs and other items are likely to produce localised reactions but jumpers, shirts and underclothes may cause large, diffuse responses which are difficult to diagnose. Christmas and birthday presents are always worth considering as likely culprits if skin problems develop shortly after those seasons.

Soap powders used to wash clothes can cause eczema if the clothes are not rinsed thoroughly. Modern detergents are extremely powerful and the products with 'biological' actions seem to be more troublesome than most.

7 Eczema confined to the hands and arms Look first of all for any tell tale limits to the skin markings. If the rash is confined to an area of skin which is in regular contact with a particular item of jewellery or with the sleeve or cuff of a jumper then a causative relationship should not be too difficult to establish.

If there aren't any telltale limits and the eczema affects the skin of the hands and arms in general then finding the irritant or allergen is likely to be more difficult. Soaps and washing powders can cause problems.

8 Eczema confined to the feet Shoes, socks and talcum powders
are the commonest causes of problems.

Many creams, ointments and other products intended for the
treatment of eczema (and other skin problems) can actually cause
or exacerbate the symptoms of eczema. Up to a third of all cases
of contact eczema may be caused or complicated by skin creams
and ointments which have either been bought over the chemist's
counter or prescribed by a doctor. You should think of this
possibility if your child's eczema seems to be getting worse
during treatment of if fresh symptoms have developed at the site
of treatment.

What can we do about it?

1 Ignore the advice and comments of seemingly well-meaning
friends and relatives. There are few diseases which attract as
much comment as eczema. Most of these comments seem
gloomy, pessimistic and intensely depressing. Ignore them.

2 Don't be too upset if you become confused by the technical
terms which are used to describe skin conditions of the
eczematous type. The truth, I'm afraid, is that doctors often
confuse themselves as well as others by using vague and
misleading terms which don't add anything to an understanding
of the condition.

3 If you can find an irritant or allergen which seems responsible
for all or part of your child's eczema then you should obviously
try and avoid contact with that substance.

4 Children who develop eczema usually suffer from dry skin. Use
a bath oil when giving your child a bath. This helps to keep water
in the skin. Use a good, plain moisturising cream twice a day and
after bathing. Moisturising creams do not add moisture to the skin
but they do help to keep moisture in the skin. If ordinary soap
makes the dryness worse then a liquid cleanser can be
substituted. Remember that too much bathing exacerbates dry
skin and that showers may be preferable.

5 Woollen clothing tends to irritate dry or eczematous skin.
Cotton clothing should be used in preference.

6 Extremes of temperature seem to be bad for eczema. Gentle
sunlight seems to help the condition.

7 Children with eczema suffer a great deal from itching. The
extent of a child's eczema depends to some extent on the amount
of itching and on the child's response. Since scratching can easily

lead to skin infection it is important to reduce the amount of itching as much as possible.

Itching can sometimes be controlled by the careful use of antihistamines and scratching can be prevented either by bandaging the eczematous area with a simple dry bandage or by giving the child cotton gloves or mittens to wear at night. Keeping the fingernails short is another obvious way to reduce the extent of the damage done by scratching.

8 Parents should touch eczematous children as often as possible. All patients with skin problems tend to feel dirty and unclean. Children who feel this way may shy away from contact with other children. Children who have eczema of any kind should, therefore, be reassured that their condition is not infectious. Regular body contact is an excellent way to provide solid reassurance.

9 Children who have eczema and who are treated as invalids may become manipulative and take advantage of their disorder. Although sympathy and treatment should be provided when required it is important not to overdo the sympathy!

10 If there is a strong family history of eczema it may be wise to control your child's diet before he develops eczema. Feeding a child on breast milk for as long as possible and withholding the introduction of eggs or dairy products can delay or prevent eczema.

11 If eczema does develop it may be worthwhile completely withdrawing eggs or dairy products from the diet for a month. If at the end of a month no improvement has been noticed then it is probably fair to say that there is unlikely to be any link. If, however, the condition of the skin has improved then I suggest that you continue to exclude the substance from the diet.

12 Children who have eczema will sometimes react abnormally to vaccines. The whooping cough vaccine should, in particular, be avoided. (See page 306 for a description of precisely when and under what conditions skin problems should be considered a contraindication to vaccination.)

13 Sweating tends to make eczema worse so avoid conditions which exacerbate sweating. Nylon clothing should be avoided. Make sure your child is never 'overdressed'.

14 Try to avoid using very strong detergents. Make sure that all clothing is thoroughly rinsed in running water.

When should we see the doctor?

It is wise to seek medical advice as soon as you notice any signs of eczema developing. There is no magical treatment available but your doctor may be able to help you decide whether or not the condition has been produced or exacerbated by an irritant or specific allergen.

What will the doctor do?

Your doctor's first task will be to attempt to identify the type of eczema.

The technique used to identify allergens is called patch testing. Suspected substances are applied quite deliberately to patches of skin in order to see if any response ensues. Patch testing is only of use for identifying allergens which produce eczema by contact with the skin.

His other main job will be to control the condition as effectively as possible. There is no certain cure available for. any form of eczema, although irritant eczema and allergic eczema may successfully be prevented if the correct irritant or allergen can be avoided.

Doctors can, however, help eczematous children in three important ways.

1 Antihistamines help stop itching. A major side effect with antihistamines is drowsiness but this problem can be used to advantage if the antihistamine is administered at night. Antihistamines are available as tablets or as medicines.

2 When eczematous conditions become infected antibiotics may be needed. Although creams and ointments containing anti-infectives are available many doctors prefer to prescribe oral anti-infectives.

3 Steroid creams and ointments are often prescribed for the treatment of eczematous skin conditions. These products improve but do not cure skin problems. They should be used with great caution since if used excessively they can exacerbate the condition rather than improve it.

A cream, by the way, is a substance with the consistency of the oily part of milk. Creams spread more easily than ointments which tend to be stickier, greasier and messier than creams. Ointments are usually preferred for very dry, crusty skin.

Epilepsy

What is it?
Epilepsy is not a single disease but is the name given to a group of disorders which produce convulsions and a loss of consciousness. Epilepsy can start at any age and epileptic fits are produced by a sudden and unusual release of electrical energy within the brain for which there is no apparent explanation. Epilepsy can be a temporary condition or a more or less permanent problem.

What causes it?
Accidents, wounds or injury can all cause epilepsy – as can excessive heat or disturbances of calcium or sugar metabolism. These factors cause epilepsy by their effect on the brain.

There is often no known cause when epilepsy develops.

What happens in an epileptic fit?
The sudden release of electrical energy within the brain can interfere with different muscles in many ways. The type and nature of symptoms produced depends upon the site and size of the electrical disturbance involved.

What different types of epileptic fit are there?
The most common and most dramatic type of epileptic fit is known as a grand mal attack or seizure. The child will suddenly go unconscious, his limbs and trunk will stiffen, and then there will be a generalised flailing and jerking of the muscles. A major epileptic fit can be very alarming for onlookers, particularly if they haven't seen one before.

Immediately prior to a grand mal attack sufferers will frequently have a strange warning sensation. They will feel that something is about to happen and they'll often cry out. This warning sensation is known as the aura. Apart from the aura a grand mal attack is very much like a febrile convulsion.

The other type of epileptic fit that most commonly affects children is the petit mal seizure. In this type of fit the child will simply lose consciousness for a few seconds. He may just seem to daydream or his attention may wander. There isn't a lot of muscle movement, as there is with a major seizure, but there may be some fluttering of the eyelids or nodding of the head.

Those are the two most common types of epileptic seizure. There are various other types of epileptic fit which can occasionally occur. For example, some children may have fits in which only one part of the body is involved (these are called Jacksonian seizures) while others may have psychomotor seizures in which the changes affect only behaviour and personality and do not produce any muscular signs.

What should we do if our child has an epileptic fit?

1 If your child has a high temperature then you should treat the fit as a febrile convulsion (see page 91).

2 If your child does not have a high temperature turn him on his side and into such a position that he will not swallow any saliva or any food he vomits. The most suitable position for an unconscious patient is described on page 5.

3 Don't try to hold him down. Don't try to put anything in his mouth or between his teeth. Don't give him anything to eat or drink.

4 Loosen any tight clothing such as a tie or belt. Undo zips and buttons where possible.

5 If your epileptic child falls do check to make sure that he has not injured himself. An epileptic child who has hit his head and who remains unconscious may have suffered a head injury.

6 Stay with your child until he has regained full consciousness. Children are sometimes confused after an epileptic fit. They may also be sleepy.

What about if our child has an aura and knows he is about to have a fit?

You won't have long – seconds rather than minutes. Simply move your child into a safe place. This should preferably be somewhere where he can lie down away from traffic and machinery or any hard objects. If possible move him into a quiet place where he won't attract a lot of spectators.

How should an epileptic child be treated?

Basically the same as any other member of the family and, as far as possible, the same as an ordinary child. Most children who have epilepsy attend normal schools. The epileptic child will need supervision while swimming. You should try and dissuade him from climbing trees or cycling on a busy road.

It is important that relatives, teachers and friends know about your child's epilepsy and that they understand, with you, that a child who is epileptic is by no means necessarily subnormal in any way. The number of successful people who have suffered from epilepsy is large. Among some of the ones most commonly quoted are Alexander the Great, Pythagoras, Julius Caesar, Napoleon, Pascal, Paganini, Dostoevsky and Edward Lear. There are very few children with epilepsy whose potential need be limited by their disease.

I have prepared a short list of tips to remember.

1 Do make sure that your child takes his medication in the right amount and at the right time. Don't make changes without consulting your doctor and don't let your child make changes either.

2 Don't give your child any over-the-counter medicine. The ingredients of such products can interfere with the medication your child is taking for his epilepsy.

3 Make an appointment to see your doctor every six months even if everything is going well. Medication levels can sometimes be reduced.

4 Children with epilepsy who are taking drugs should wear identification bracelets such as Medic-Alert.

5 Eating too little or going to bed too late can induce epilepsy.

6 It's better not to have a lock on the bathroom or lavatory door.

How do we make the diagnosis?

There are a number of disorders which can be mistaken for epilepsy. A febrile convulsion (see page 90) is probably the condition most commonly confused with an epileptic attack. Febrile convulsions occur only when a child has a high temperature. They are not usually preceded by an aura. However, if your child has a fit then you should allow a doctor to make the diagnosis. You certainly should not simply put it down as febrile convulsion and ignore it.

When should we call the doctor?

If your child has had a fit you should call for medical help as soon as possible unless you are already aware that your child has epileptic fits and you are satisfied that the most recent fit was no longer, no deeper and no different to previous fits.

There is not usually any need to call an ambulance unless the fit lasts for more than five or ten minutes.

Can epilepsy be inherited?
Yes. There is a small risk that in some cases epilepsy can be inherited. Ask your doctor if you are in any doubt. He may arrange a referral to a geneticist if you are planning further additions to your family.

What will the doctor do?
To begin with he will, of course, want to make sure that your child is indeed suffering from epilepsy. He will probably arrange for a full neurological examination to be done by a hospital neurologist. Blood tests and an electroencephalogram will probably be done.

Once the diagnosis has been confirmed then your doctor will begin treatment with one or more anti-convulsant drugs. Two things must be said about these drugs. First, there is no effective anti-convulsant drug available which does not ever cause side effects. Drowsiness is one of the commonest side effects. Second, it usually takes some time to find the most suitable dose of an anti-convulsant drug. The treatment will probably have to be altered each time a fit occurs with the dose being increased if fits continue or decreased if side effects develop.

Fainting

What is it?
Fainting is a temporary loss of consciousness caused by a part of the nervous system which is outside voluntary control.

Just before he goes unconscious a child may feel light headed and slightly nauseous. He will probably be pale and clammy and may have a glazed look in his eyes.

Fainting attacks occur in girls more than boys and are rare in children under the age of 10.

What causes it?
Fainting is produced by a reduction in the blood flow to the brain.

The brain needs a good supply of oxygenated blood in order to function effectively and when it is deprived of blood it needs protecting. An individual who faints will fall down into a horizontal position, gravity will consequently be less of a problem and the blood flow to the brain will be easier to restore and maintain.

That's the physiological explanation of fainting. In practice, of course, there seem to be many possible causes. Sometimes a child who is standing in a crowd will faint, particularly if the atmosphere is rather hot and stuffy. A low blood sugar can make fainting more likely so children commonly faint in morning assembly at school when they haven't had a proper breakfast. Suddenly changing position is another cause. The child who jumps up out of a chair or out of bed is quite likely to faint. Sometimes the faint may be partial, with the victim merely feeling light-headed and dizzy but managing to stay conscious.

The other major cause of fainting is anxiety. There is no doubt that this is the factor which often links together the mass fainting sessions which occasionally occur at such varied centres as school assembly halls and pop music concerts.

What is the difference between a faint and a fit?

A child who has a faint will usually drift quietly and gently into unconsciousness. Afterwards he will remember things slowly going black or going round and round. The child who has had a fit is more likely to have convulsions and signs of muscular disorder. Afterwards the child who has had a fit will probably not remember anything.

The child who faints doesn't usually wet himself whereas the child who has a fit may do. The child who faints will usually make a very full and speedy recovery. The child who has a fit will probably sleep afterwards.

What can we do about it?

The only risk with fainting is that the child may injure himself as he falls and so a child who says he feels faint should be laid down flat as soon as possible. Any tight clothing should be loosened and the child should be left to rest as quietly as possible. Consciousness will return when the blood flow to the brain is restored. If this isn't possible it usually helps to get the child to put his head down between his knees. While he is in that position put your hand on the back of his head and get him to try and stand up. The effort will push blood into the brain quickly.

The child who has regular mid-morning fainting attacks

probably needs more to eat at breakfast time.

When do we need to see the doctor?

You don't need to see the doctor about an isolated faint. You need medical advice only if the fainting recurs or if you are uncertain about whether your child has fainted or had a fit.

If a child faints and doesn't come round within two or three minutes then you should call the doctor straightaway.

What will the doctor do?

If he is convinced that your child has simply fainted the doctor is unlikely to do anything. If he is uncertain about whether or not your child is fainting or fitting he will probably arrange for an electroencephalogram to be done.

Fever

What is it?

The normal temperature within the human body is 98.6 degrees Fahrenheit (37 degrees centigrade). When the temperature rises above this the child is said to have a fever. A fever is not an illness. It is a symptom.

What causes it?

A sophisticated defence system within the human body helps to maintain the body's temperature at a steady level. The amount of heat produced by the body's own metabolic processes is matched with the amount of heat lost through the skin.

Although their temperature regulating mechanism is not fully efficient children can usually cope with quite considerable variations in the external temperature by regulating the loss of heat from the body. The child who is in a hot room will start to sweat, and his superficial blood vessels will dilate so that the blood flow through the skin is increased. Sweating gets rid of heat because as the fluid evaporates from the skin it takes heat with it. The dilation of superficial blood vessels gets rid of heat since the more warm blood there is in close contact with the environment the greater will be the amount of heat that is lost.

On the other hand the child who is in a cold room will shiver and his blood vessels will constrict where they pass through the skin. Shivering produces heat because it initiates muscle action. Shutting down some of the superficial blood vessels preserves body heat by minimising the amount of heat lost through the blood in the skin.

These temperature control mechanisms can fail for several different reasons. They can fail if the external temperature falls too low or gets too high for the body's own control mechanism to be able to cope. More common than this, however, are those occasions when the body's temperature control is disturbed from inside rather than outside. If your child has an infectious disease which interferes with the body's metabolic processes and produces extra body heat then the body temperature may rise. Because the temperature control mechanism in children is far more sensitive than it is in adults a relatively inoffensive infectious disease may produce a fairly dramatic change in body temperature.

Is a fever always dangerous?

No. There is now evidence which suggests that when the body temperature rises in response to some internal infection it is a planned rather than an unplanned response and that the high internal temperature will help speed recovery, presumably by creating an internal environment which the infective organisms find unfavourable.

Only if the fever rises too high or too quickly does it pose serious problems.

How do we measure a fever?

The traditional way to tell whether or not a child is running a high temperature is to place the back of the hand on to the child's forehead. But a fascinating piece of research done at the Johns Hopkins Hospital in America showed that even well-trained nurses have difficulty in judging a child's temperature by using their own hands. In a project which involved over a thousand children a team of nurses mistakenly thought that 42 per cent of those with fevers had got normal temperatures.

The hand on the forehead is probably better than nothing but the thermometer is the obvious instrument to use. It really isn't as difficult to handle as a lot of parents seem to think. The temperature can be taken in any one of three places: in the mouth, under the armpit or in the rectum. You must take the temperature in the same place each time you take it during a particular illness. This isn't for reasons of hygiene (I'm assuming that you're going to wash the thermometer every time you've used it) but is for the important reason that the body temperature in those three sites varies very slightly.

The best place to take a child's temperature is in the armpit. He isn't likely to swallow it or sit on it there. Place the thermometer in the bare armpit and hold it there for two minutes.

To make sure that the thermometer does not fall out of place bring the child's arm across his chest and tell him to hold his opposite shoulder.

Before you take the temperature you should put your thermometer into cold water and leave it there for a minute. Dry it carefully and make sure you can read the position of the mercury easily enough. Twiddle the thermometer around in your fingers until you can see the mercury or alcohol level. Don't, incidentally, take a child's temperature if he is nursing a hot-water bottle or if he has just had a hot drink.

After you've taken the temperature put the thermometer into a little liquid antiseptic so that it will be ready for use next time.

When is a fever too high?

The 'normal' body temperature is 98.6 degrees Fahrenheit but in practice the body temperature will often vary by a degree or two at different times of the day. The body's temperature is usually at its highest in the late afternoon and at its lowest at about 4 a.m. in the morning when the whole range of body functions are just ticking over. Temperature can also rise as a result of exercise.

Your child has a genuine fever if his temperature is over 100.4 degrees Fahrenheit (38 degrees centigrade), isn't wearing too many clothes and hasn't just come in after a period of hectic exercise.

How can we tell if our child's temperature is rising too fast?

The rate at which a fever rises is important because if the temperature goes up too quickly your child may have a febrile convulsion. If your child's temperature is above 100.4 degrees Fahrenheit and after a four-hour interval it has risen by more than 0.5 degrees then you should try to reduce the temperature and slow down the rate at which it is rising by tepid sponging, by taking clothes off your child and by opening a window.

Is sweating of any significance?

Sweating is a mechanism used by the body to help reduce the body temperature. If your child has been playing outside and has become overheated then he will sweat. As the sweat evaporates from the skin it will take with it body heat.

When your child has an infection things are rather different. The body's thermostat which regulates all the temperature control mechanisms is altered by the release of special chemicals, themselves produced by the body's reaction to the invading organisms which are responsible for the infection.

These chemicals set the thermostat a little higher so that it is your child's own body which produces the high temperature and the accompanying sweating.

If your child has been overexercising or has got over excited and he's sweating then his body temperature is probably rising and the sweating mechanism is being brought into action to counteract that effect. If, on the other hand, your child has got an infection and he is sweating then it may be that his temperature is falling.

What can we do about a fever?

1 Do not make the mistake of wrapping up a child who is hot. Do that and you'll simply send his temperature soaring even higher. The child who is hot needs fewer clothes, not more.

2 Sponging with tepid water or even warm water will help to reduce the temperature. Do not use cold water because if you do you'll reduce the superficial blood circulation and send the temperature up instead of bringing it down. You don't need to tepid sponge unless the temperature is above 102 degrees Fahrenheit or is rising rapidly.

3 If your child's temperature is 102 degrees Fahrenheit or over and he appears unwell then you can bring down the temperature a little by using aspirin or paracetamol. (See bottle label for dosages.) There is no need to use drugs to bring down a child's temperature if he seems well. There is no evidence to suggest that by bringing the temperature down your child will get better quicker.

4 One of the main risks with a fever is that your child will become dehydrated. Do, therefore, ensure that he takes plenty of fluids. Food doesn't matter.

5 If your child wants to stay in bed then let him. But if he wants to get up there is no reason why you should keep him in bed.

When should we ask for medical advice?
1 If your child appears particularly or persistently unwell.
2 If the temperature is rising rapidly and you cannot control it.
3 If your child has a past history of febrile convulsions and his temperature is rising uncontrollably.
4 If the fever is above 102 degrees Fahrenheit.
5 As a good general rule any child who wants to stay in bed should be seen by a doctor.

What will the doctor do?
He will try and decide why your child has a fever. If he thinks the fever is caused by an infection then he will probably prescribe a suitable antibiotic. It is important to make sure that any prescribed antibiotic is given as a complete course. Don't stop giving the drug just because the temperature has fallen because if you do the infection is likely to return.

Flat feet

What are they?
When a baby is born its feet are quite flat. As the baby grows and learns to walk unaided arches develop on the inner edges of the feet. These arches are formed as the muscles of the feet and legs develop in strength and the fatty pads which normally fill in this area slowly disappear. Arches don't usually appear until a child reaches the age of 3 or 4 years.

If those arches do not develop properly for any reason then your child will have flat feet. This condition is by no means as common as many parents and some doctors suspect.

How do we make the diagnosis?
You shouldn't make a diagnosis of 'flat feet' or 'flat foot' until your child is 4 years old. The arches are still developing until that time and so any such diagnosis would be quite premature. At that age you can best judge whether or not your child has flat feet by getting him to stand on tip toes. You should then be able to see an arch developing even if one wasn't obviously present when your child was standing with his feet flat on the ground.

It is sometimes said that the diagnosis of flat feet can be made by looking at the shoes to see where the greatest amount of wear has taken place. I'm not sure that this is as good an idea as looking at the feet but if your child wears down the heels and soles of his shoes on the inner side then there may be a problem. Another trick is to get the child to stand in water and then put his feet on to a plain piece of paper. If the feet are of a normal shape the footprints will show a classic 'footprint' pattern but if the feet are flat then the whole foot will leave an outline on the paper.

If a child complains of pains in his feet after modest exercise then a diagnosis of flat feet is certainly worth consideration.

How do we stop flat feet developing?
To encourage the feet to develop properly encourage your child to walk about in bare feet as often as possible.

Ensure that when shoes are worn they fit well and provide good support. Children who spend too much time in tennis shoes or pumps may complain of aching feet. If this is the case it is clearly a good idea to buy something which offers more support. If the feet are to develop properly shoes should not cramp or pinch. I have given some notes on shoe buying on page 286.

What can we do about it?
First of all you can stop worrying. Only about 5 per cent of all children who are diagnosed as having flat feet grow up with flat feet.

Exercises are sometimes suggested as an aid to building up the muscles of the feet and improving the shape of the arch.

Such exercises won't definitely help but they won't do any harm so you can, if you like, persuade your child to try simple daily exercises. Standing on tip toes for a few minutes or raising and lowering from tip toe to flat feet a dozen times a day might well help.

The most useful way to help a child who definitely has flat feet is to provide shoes with what is known as an 'inner raise'. A small extra piece of leather is tacked on to the heel of the child's shoes to increase the height of the heel at that point by no more than three-sixteenths of an inch. This must be done by a professional and not just tacked on haphazardly at home. An inner raise will help your child to acquire a better walking habit and a better arch within a couple of years. These raises are not usually necessary after the child reaches the age of 9.

When do we need to see the doctor?
The great majority of children whose parents think they have flat feet don't actually have flat feet at all. The majority of children who do have flat feet will eventually acquire foot arches without anyone interfering.

Having said that I recognise that this is a subject which worries many parents. I suggest that if you are still concerned about your child's feet you should visit your doctor for advice and reassurance. If you are contemplating having your child's shoes fitted with an inner raise visit your doctor anyway.

If a child's feet are obviously deformed in any way, or if they are painful when the child has walked a short distance or taken modest exercise then a visit to the doctor is indicated.

What will the doctor do?
If he thinks that there is any real problem he will probably arrange an appointment with an orthopaedic surgeon who will examine and possibly X-ray your child's feet.

Food allergy

What is it?
In the same way that some individuals are allergic to pollen, feathers or cats, so some are allergic to specific types of food. Food allergies are extremely common and are responsible for a wide range of symptoms and specific diseases.

What causes it?
The food responsible for the allergy produces symptoms by having a direct effect on the body's immunological defences. Sometimes a food that has been eaten before only rarely will produce violent symptoms. Occasionally a food that has been eaten quite regularly will suddenly produce severe symptoms. More commonly a food to which an individual is allergic will produce relatively mild symptoms which are not immediately recognised as being produced by food.

What symptoms and disorders are caused by food allergy?
Individuals who are allergic to food may produce an enormous
range of different symptoms and signs. I've prepared a list of
some of the commonest physical and mental problems known to
be associated with food allergy.

1 Migraine.
2 Asthma.
3 Eczema.
4 Anxiety.
5 Palpitations.
6 Behavioural problems.
7 Aphthous ulcers and mouth sores.
8 Skin rashes.
9 Rhinitis.
10 Abdominal pains.
11 Diarrhoea.
12 Bedwetting.
13 Joint pains.
14 Depression.
15 Tiredness and general lethargy.
16 Obesity.
17 Vomiting.

What foods most commonly cause symptoms?
1 Cows' milk.
2 Wheat.
3 Oranges.
4 Eggs.
5 Tea and coffee.
6 Chocolate.
7 Beef.
8 Yeast.
9 Cane sugar.
10 Mushrooms.
11 Peas.
12 Corn.
13 Peanuts.
14 Rice.
15 Pork.
16 Tomatoes.
17 Apples.

18 Cheese.
19 Fish.
20 Artificial colours and preservatives.

How do we make the diagnosis?

It isn't always easy to make a firm diagnosis of a food allergy. Often the diagnosis is only made when symptoms and signs persist and all other possible explanations have been investigated and abandoned. You should suspect a food allergy in the following circumstances.

1 If you notice any correlation between your child's symptoms and any particular foodstuffs. If, for example, you notice that your child always falls ill on a particular day then a little investigation may show that particular types of food are eaten on that day.
2 If a child is known to have other allergies – for example hay fever – then he is more likely to suffer from a food allergy than other children.
3 Occasionally children who suffer from a food allergy may be able to disguise their symptoms by repeated eating of the food in question. This is known as masking. If your child shows a very strong liking for one particular foodstuff then he may be allergic to that food.
4 If the food a child is allergic to is high in calories then 'masking' can lead to obesity.
5 Sometimes a child may develop very dramatic symptoms after eating a food to which he is allergic. A generalised swollen, red, itchy rash suggests a fierce allergy reaction.

What can we do about it?

1 A child can develop a serious and dangerous allergy reaction to food. Keep your child away from any food to which he has already exhibited any obvious and dramatic allergy.
2 When there is a strong family history of allergy reactions developing it is wise to breast feed a new baby for six months. There is good evidence to show that if a baby receives only breast milk for this period the risk of allergy reactions developing is much reduced.
3 Whenever a child develops an allergy problem of any kind it is worthwhile thinking of a food allergy as a possible cause. Eggs and milk are two of the commonest food allergens. If, for

example, a child develops eczema then it is a good idea to omit one of these items from the diet for two or three weeks. If at the end of that time there has been a noticeable improvement in the condition then the item can be kept out of the diet permanently. If the improvement is slight or not noticeable then the item can be restored to the diet. If restoring the item to the diet produces a deterioration in the condition then a link can be regarded as having been identified. If there is no deterioration after a five-day interval then another possible food allergen can be tested.

4 Once a food allergen has been identified the only solution is to avoid it and all foodstuffs which may contain it. As children grow, however, they often lose their allergy to food. After a period of a year identified food allergens can be reintroduced into the diet in small quantities. If no symptoms ensue then the food can be restored to the diet.

When do we need the doctor?

If you suspect that your child may be allergic to a food but you don't know what then you should ask your doctor for help. If your own family doctor doesn't deal with allergy problems himself then he will be able to arrange the appropriate referral to an allergy specialist.

What will the doctor do?

One of the most effective ways to identify a food allergen is to put a child on an exclusion diet. For five days the patient is fed on nothing but foods known to be extremely unlikely to produce allergy symptoms. Lamb meat products, fresh pears and bottled spring water are three commonly used foods. In the weeks which follow all the possible food allergens are then introduced into the diet individually. It is usually then possible to identify the food to which a patient is allergic by the reappearance of symptoms. Although this technique could be used by parents alone I think it should be reserved for use under expert supervision. It is important to ensure that a child's dietary intake is not badly disordered during the testing and expert advice is often needed to find out which foodstuffs contain what additives.

Antihistamines can be used to help control symptoms and some doctors are experimenting with desensitising injections prepared from minute quantities of food allergens but the only real way a doctor can help is by assisting you to identify the food allergen. Once that has been done the answer is simply to avoid that food.

German measles

What is it?
A very common infectious disease caused by a virus. Also known as rubella.

How do we make the diagnosis?
Children with german measles usually begin with the symptoms of a cold. They also often complain of tenderness behind the ears and at the back of the neck. The typical rash of german measles starts behind the ears and on the face and then spreads all over the body. To begin with small flat pink spots are visible but later on these clump together to form red patches. There may be a little itching but there isn't usually any noticeable fever.

Is it catching?
German measles is fairly infectious. After contact with an infected person it may take three weeks for symptoms to develop. The child who has been in contact and who has contracted german measles is infectious from one day before the appearance of the rash until two days after it has gone.

What can we do about it?
There is no cure for german measles and there is not usually any need for symptomatic treatment. An effective vaccine is available and all girls approaching puberty should be vaccinated because of the risks involved when pregnant women catch german measles. For this same reason it is important to keep any infected child away from any woman who may be pregnant.

What's the truth about german measles and pregnant women?
If a woman who is pregnant becomes infected with german measles she may have a miscarriage and lose her baby or she may give birth to a congenitally deformed baby. Babies born to women who have been in contact with german measles may, for example, be born blind, deaf or with heart problems. The first

three months of a pregnancy are the most dangerous as far as german measles is concerned but the infection is best avoided by all expectant mothers.

Any woman who is hoping to become pregnant can have a blood test done to find out whether or not she is immune to german measles. If she isn't then she would be wise to have the vaccination. Any woman who is pregnant can also have the test and if the result suggests that she has contracted the infection during her pregnancy an injection of gamma globulin may be recommended.

When do we need to see the doctor?

Complications are relatively rare with german measles but problems to watch out for include vomiting, earache and headache. Any unexpected symptom merits a call to the doctor.

Habits

What are they?

We all have habits. We depend on them to help us get through life without forever having to remember to do things. Cleaning your teeth every morning and every evening is a habit that is useful. Habits only become a problem when they involve a child in some action that is harmful, antisocial or annoying.

In this section I intend to deal only with those habits that are in some way harmful or disruptive. Habits which fit into these categories are sometimes known as 'behavioural problems.'

What sort of habits cause problems?

It is impossible to prepare a completely comprehensive list of all the habits that worry parents. I have, however, prepared a list of some of the commonest.

1 Thumb sucking Young babies are born with a natural inclination to suck things which seem the right shape, size and texture. It is this inclination to suck which ensures that a baby takes to his mother's breast shortly after he is born. A baby's thumb, or indeed, any of his fingers, is not all that different to a maternal nipple and thumb sucking is, therefore, a natural habit.

Most young children give up thumb sucking when they reach the age of 3 or 4 years.

Two things to watch for when a baby, infant or young child sucks his thumb are that he is getting enough love and attention and that, if he is being breast fed, he is getting long enough at the breast. If he's losing weight as well as sucking his thumb then he probably needs to spend more time sucking a nipple and less time sucking a thumb.

Thumb sucking is only really a problem if it produces actual damage to the skin of the thumb (if it does then you should make sure that the skin is kept clean) or if it persists after the age of 6 years. After that age it can push the teeth forward and so should be discouraged as much as possible.

Do not, however, get too excited about thumb sucking. If you turn the problem into a major battle between yourself and your child then you'll probably produce a great deal of anger and resentment. You may even turn your baby into a 'secret sucker'. Ignore it as much as you can.

2 Dummy sucking Babies and young children suck dummies for the same reason that they suck their thumbs – they find it soothing and comforting. There isn't really any difference between the two habits although the risks to the thumb itself and to the teeth are obviously less. If a baby does suck a dummy then it is important to make sure that it is kept clean. It really is rather unhygienic to allow passers-by to put a dummy back into a pram when it has been tossed on to the pavement.

On balance, I think that thumb sucking is probably less hazardous than dummy sucking.

3 Temper tantrum These are sometimes rather frightening but they are very common in babies and small children. Most young children have at least one temper tantrum in their life. Children have temper tantrums because they are unhappy, cross or frustrated. If you think that your child is justifiably unhappy, cross or frustrated then you should do what you can to remedy the situation. If, however, you feel that your child is behaving unreasonably then you should take no notice of the tantrum. The child who learns that he can get his own way by throwing a tantrum will continue to do it. The child whose tantrum is ignored will give up the habit before it becomes a problem.

4 Sleep walking Although they don't walk with their arms stretched out in front of them as a lot of people imagine, children who sleep walk really do wander around while still asleep. Their eyes may be open and they may seem awake but if they meet someone they know very well they won't appear to notice them. Children usually sleep walk because they are worried about something at home or at school. Don't make a fuss about the sleep walking but try and find out if there is something causing your child to worry.

It's best not to wake a sleep walking child. Just lead him back to bed gently. I do not believe in old wives' tales which suggest that you put a tray full of water by the bedside. I think that is rather cruel and quite likely to do more harm than good.

5 Head banging Head banging sometimes occurs in mentally retarded children who are bored or who don't have enough to do. It can, however, often be a manipulative exercise employed by perfectly alert and intelligent children who want to get their own way. It is a variation on the temper tantrum theme. Move your child to a room or position where he can't do himself any harm but take as little notice as you can. You certainly should not give in to a child who uses head banging in an attempt to get his own way.

6 Masturbation Despite all the ancient theories about this causing blindness and mental illness masturbation is a perfectly natural phenomenon and is a normal part of a child's growing up. A child can masturbate as much as he wants without going short-sighted, let alone blind.

7 Unusual eating habits Most children will eat or drink strange things if given the chance. It isn't anything to worry about unless they happen to eat something poisonous! Picking up bits of soap, coal or dirt and trying them for taste is just a normal part of growing up. Children are naturally and incurably curious. Knowing that this habit is a natural one you should ensure that all potential poisons are kept well out of reach or locked up.

8 Sexual exploration It is quite natural for children to be interested in their own sexual organs and the sexual organs of other children. Do not be distressed if you repeatedly find your child playing with or investigating his own sexual apparatus or that of other children. Only if the interest becomes obsessional or unnatural should you seek professional advice.

9 Lying It is difficult to draw distinct lines about when lying is a punishable offence or merely a part of growing up. On the whole, however, I think it is fair to accept a child's lies as natural unless they are designed to cover up a sequence of misdeeds. An occasional lie, designed to cover up a behavioural error, needs only to be punished. Repeated lying may merit professional advice. It is important to differentiate between lies and imagination, by the way. Children invariably make up stories and elaborate events. This isn't anything to worry about unless the child's imagination takes over from reality.

10 Stealing Small children often steal because they do not properly appreciate the meaning and implication of 'ownership'. When they 'borrow' other children's toys they should be gently encouraged to understand the concept of ownership.

Children who understand that stealing is wrong still do it for one of three main reasons. They steal because they genuinely think they need whatever it is they take. They steal because their friends and peers steal and they don't want to be left out or considered 'chicken'. Or they steal because they desperately need to draw attention to their emotional needs. Habitual stealing does often fall into this last category.

If your child makes a habit of stealing then you should ask yourself which of these reasons is the right one.

11 Soiling Even in older children occasional soiling is nothing to worry about. Paradoxically the most common cause is constipation with overflow diarrhoea and the solution is to deal with the constipation. Soiling is usually made worse by embarrassment or punishment so offer your child encouragement and support rather than threats and anger.

12 Destructive behaviour It is quite natural for a child to break toys occasionally in fits of anger or temper. It is more worrying when a child consistently destroys his own toys or toys belonging to other children. This sort of behaviour usually implies an emotional problem which may need sorting out with professional help.

13 Object attachment Many small children become very much attached to particular dolls, teddy bears or blankets! There doesn't seem to be any particular significance to these 'comfort' objects and children invariably grow out of their attachment by the age of about 10 years. There isn't any need to deliberately try to break a child's attachment to any particular object. This usually happens quite naturally and slowly with the once-favoured object gradually being left more and more on one side. It may be sought out for comfort well into the teenage years but this isn't any cause for real concern.

14 Bedwetting This is discussed on page 40.
15 Crying This is discussed on page 98.
16 Breath holding This is discussed on page 60.
17 Phobias This is discussed on page 204.
18 Sleeplessness This is discussed on page 213.
19 Overactivity This is discussed on page 197.
20 Hiccups This is discussed on page 158.
21 Bad habits are discussed on page 293.

What can we do about it?
If your child has a habit which worries you then you will usually find that the habit will disappear quicker if you take little notice and do not allow your child to know that you are worried. It also helps to praise your child when he isn't doing whatever it is you find objectionable rather than to threaten or punish him when he is doing it. Support and encouragement and other positive actions are far more effective than threats and punishments.

Remember that many of these unwanted habits develop because a child is under too much pressure or stress. I have described the sort of ways that stress can be produced on page 288 where I have also discussed possible solutions.

When do we need the doctor?
If after reading the relevant material in this section you are still worried about your child's habit then you should seek medical advice. Your doctor will be able to tell you whether your child's

behaviour falls within normal limits or if specialist advice should be sought.

Hay fever

What is it?

Hay fever is an allergy reaction – usually to pollen – and the symptoms which develop are merely an exaggerated part of the body's defence mechanism. The body reacts to the pollen as though it were a dangerous threat and does all it can to oppose its presence. The eyes are irritated and they water a good deal to help wash away the pollen. The pollen that gets into the nose produces sneezing and a copious amount of nasal fluid.

Since the pollen which produces these symptoms is produced seasonally this disorder is very much a seasonal problem.

What causes it?

A large variety of different types of pollen can cause hay fever. Individual patients usually become hypersensitive to one type of pollen and so complain of symptoms during the period when that particular plant or tree is producing pollen. Children who suffer from hay fever in April or May are usually sensitive to tree pollen (plane trees and silver birch trees seem to be popular culprits) while children whose symptoms appear in June and July are usually sensitive to grass or nettle pollen.

How do we make the diagnosis?

If your child seems to have the symptoms of a common cold every spring or summer then he probably has hay fever. A streaming nose, itchy eyes or incessant sneezing during the months of April, May, June or July means that hay fever is a pretty safe diagnosis.

Children with hay fever sometimes also complain of having a blocked nose and a diminished sense of smell. The blocked nose may result in regular mouth breathing and that can mean that the patient wakes every morning with a dry, irritable throat. If fluid trickles down the back of the throat in the night the patient may wake up coughing – this problem is called post-nasal drip.

Hay fever can start at any age but in more than 80 per cent of cases it starts between the ages of 5 and 25. Boys seem to suffer more than girls.

Should the symptoms occur outside the April-July period then the chances are that the cause is some non-seasonal allergen. Perennial allergic rhinitis, as it is called, can be caused by feather pillows, house dust, animals, foods, cooking fumes, cigarette smoke and even medicines. Apart from the absence of a seasonal factor the main difference between a hay fever and perennial rhinitis is that the symptoms of hay fever tend to be more severe – with very violent episodes and eyes which weep so much that the patient finds it difficult to see.

Is it inherited?
Yes. Like all allergy problems hay fever can be inherited.

What can we do about it?
1 It is obviously wise to keep your child away from the problem pollen as much as possible. This means keeping house doors and windows closed during the summer months and keeping the car windows shut too while travelling. It's wise not to allow sufferers to go for walks in areas where there is long grass.
2 Children who suffer most from eye symptoms sometimes benefit from wearing dark glasses. These help keep the pollen out of the eyes.
3 There is a psychological element to hay fever. The child who is worried or anxious will suffer more.
4 If you're travelling abroad you should remember that it is possible for a child to suffer from hay fever for longer than usual. Hay fever symptoms start when pollen is being reproduced. The hay fever season in Southern Europe begins at the start of April. In some parts of the United States of America the hay fever season begins in August.
5 Hay fever symptoms usually seem less dramatic on the coast. Seaside holidays are probably better than country holidays for young children who suffer from hay fever.
6 Many newspapers print pollen counts but these are at the moment of rather questionable value. Pollen counts vary a good deal and reports of the previous day's count are therefore of limited use. Attempts to forecast pollen counts depend upon the availability of accurate information from meteorologists and unfortunately such information is not often available.

7 Hay fever is a disorder which is often regarded as something more comical than serious. However, if the pollen which causes the hay fever goes further down the respiratory tract your child may cough, wheeze and get short of breath. There is an association between hay fever and asthma but it is important to remember that the child who has got hay fever won't necessarily get asthma. Since there is a link between all allergic problems there is also a chance that the child with hay fever may also suffer from eczema.

8 Hay fever can be a dreadful nuisance for older children taking school examinations which usually seem to be organised to match the worst of the hay fever season. It may be worth asking for special care and for a doctor's letter if a child suffers a good deal.

9 Hay fever usually seems to be worst early in the morning and then again in the evening. It is least troublesome in the middle of the day. It is particularly important to keep windows and doors shut at both ends of the day.

10 Remember that while rain early in the pollen season tends to promote grass growth and make hay fever worse, rain during the middle of the pollen season reduces symptoms by preventing the release of pollen.

When do we need the doctor?

If your child suffers only mild inconvenience or if you can control the hay fever symptoms by limiting his exposure to pollen then there is little point in seeking medical advice. If, however, the hay fever symptoms are severely incapacitating or there is some special circumstance (for example, the taking of an examination) then a visit to the doctor can be useful.

What will the doctor do?

There are a variety of alternatives available for your doctor to try.

1 The first drug to be tried is usually an antihistamine. The symptoms of hay fever are produced by the action of a substance called histamine on blood vessels, mucous glands and muscle. Antihistamines, as you might suspect, oppose this action. Antihistamines are often very effective and extremely useful. They are available as tablets for patients who have general hay fever symptoms, as eye drops for patients whose problems are mainly confined to their eyes, and as nasal drops for patients whose symptoms are mainly restricted to sneezing and a runny nose. Antihistamines do cause drowsiness but this side effect can usually be avoided by trial and error. There are dozens of different antihistamines available and although one product in this group may cause severe drowsiness another may not. Your doctor will probably experiment until he finds a suitable brand.

2 Products which contain sodium cromoglycate are useful in the prevention of hay fever. Available as drops and sprays, this drug needs to be used regularly if it is to be effective. Sodium cromoglycate works by preventing the production of histamine.

3 Steroid drugs are extremely powerful and can be used as eye drops, nasal sprays, tablets or long-lasting 'depot' injections. These drugs will relieve the symptoms of hay fever and may prevent the development of symptoms. There are risks associated with the use of steroid drugs since these are capable of suppressing some of the body's own hormone production.

4 Decongestants are sometimes used when hay fever has produced congestion and stuffiness. These drugs, usually available as nose drops, may provide temporary relief but it is important not to use them for too long. If used excessively decongestants can produce rebound congestion.

5 Doctors will sometimes arrange skin tests in an attempt to find the precise cause of a patient's allergy. Once the nature of the allergy has been determined desensitising injections may be arranged. Minute but steadily increasing doses of the allergen responsible for the patient's symptoms are injected. Courses of injections vary from three jabs to as many as eighteen. These usually have to be begun several months before the hay fever season is due to start. On average eight or nine injections are given at weekly intervals. These injections then have to be given in subsequent years if the full benefit is to be obtained. After having the injection for three years three quarters of all patients treated will notice some improvement. Of the patients who do gain benefit only a third will notice a really marked improvement. A good many doctors believe that the advantages to be gained by using desensitising injections do not always outweigh the disadvantages. Since the injections do contain the very allergen to which the patient is sensitive a reaction may follow an injection. The reaction may be quite serious and for this reason most doctors like patients to remain nearby for half an hour after each injection has been given. Clearly the hay fever symptoms have to be very bad to contemplate such a form of treatment.

Head injury

When do we need to see the doctor?
You must see a doctor without delay if, after a head injury, your child:
1 Loses consciousness even if only for a few moments.
2 Vomits.
3 Seems exceptionally drowsy.
4 Complains of an ache or pain in the head.
5 Loses blood from his nose, mouth or ears.
6 Loses any watery fluid from his nose or ears.
7 Has any injury to the scalp which might suggest the possibility of an injury to the bone. A cut or gash on the scalp usually requires quite a heavy knock and that sort of injury can also cause an injury to the skull bones. Scalp wounds tend to bleed a lot, by the way, because the scalp tissues are well supplied with blood vessels.

What can we do?
You can stop any bleeding by pressing hard on the site. If the child is also unconscious you should look after the child as recommended on page 5.

What will the doctor do?
In addition to repairing any obvious, superficial wounds the doctor will, if he thinks it is necessary, arrange for X-ray pictures to be taken of the child's skull. It is important to remember that X-ray photographs are not always necessary after a bone injury. Because head injuries are difficult to assess a child with an injury of this type may be kept in hospital overnight for 'observation'. This means exactly what it says and nothing more.

Headache

What causes it?
Headache is a fairly common symptom in small children. It is rather more common in older children. Although it is usually caused by a minor problem it should always be taken seriously.

The cause which must always be borne in mind is, of course, an injury to the head. This is discussed above.

If there has been no recent injury there are a number of other possible explanations for a headache. The cause which most parents fear is probably a brain tumour but in practice this is an exceedingly rare problem. One recent survey showed that out of 1000 patients who were referred to a specialist for investigations of headaches only one brain tumour was found. That was a series of patients selected and referred from among those seen by general practitioners!

Stress is a much more common cause of headache, even in young children. Recurring headaches caused by anxiety will often be accompanied by other signs of nervousness such as tics, tremors, difficulty in getting to sleep and a poor appetite. Sometimes stress headaches occur only on certain days of the week when a child has to attend certain classes or meet specific people.

Catarrh and sinus troubles are also common causes of headache. When a headache follows a cold, is accompanied by a feeling of stuffiness and seems worse across the front of the head then catarrh must be considered as a very possible cause.

When the headache is accompanied by other symptoms such as fever, vomiting, neck stiffness and irritability then meningitis must be considered as a possible cause. This is a serious condition in which the brain's covering (the meninges) is infected. Meningitis can follow some childhood infections and although it is not a common disorder it must always be considered when a child has a headache. In addition to meningitis infections fevers of other kinds can cause headaches, possibly because the fever that accompanies an infection produces dehydration.

Migraine is a problem which doesn't affect children as often as adults, but it is still worth keeping in mind. Migraine attacks tend to be recurrent, they tend to be accompanied by vomiting and they often seem to be triggered by some specific factor. I've discussed migraine in children at greater length on page 180.

Tension headaches develop because the muscles around the head are kept taut and are not allowed to relax. Trying to read in a bad light is a common cause of headaches around the eyes and across the forehead. The eyes aren't damaged by reading in bad light, by the way, it's just that the reader tends to screw up his eyes in order to concentrate. And screwing up the muscles eventually produces pain. Putting a better light in is the best way to prevent this headache from recurring.

Earache and toothache (see pages 117 and 234 respectively) can also cause pains in the head while epilepsy and high blood pressure are two of the less common causes of headache. Constipation isn't really likely to be directly responsible for the development of a headache.

What can we do about it?

If putting your child in a dark room, offering reassurance and giving aspirin or paracetamol doesn't relieve the headache in an hour or two then you should ask for medical advice. If headaches are accompanied by any other symptoms such as vomiting, fever, neck stiffness and lack of consciousness then you should call your doctor without any delay. And if the headache follows a head injury then you should get immediate advice.

If headaches recur it is wise to try and find out whether or not there is any responsible factor which you can deal with yourself. You may be able to solve a problem at school, for example, without too much difficulty. A quiet word with the appropriate schoolteacher may be all that is needed.

What will the doctor do?

Medical treatment will depend upon the cause. Infections need to be treated with antibiotics. In some cases skull X-rays may be taken although the great majority of skull X-rays show no abnormality. Lumbar punctures may have to be done to exclude meningitis.

Heat exhaustion

What is it?

In very hot and humid conditions when the body sweats a good deal the loss of fluids and salt can cause exhaustion, cramps, pallor, nausea, rapid breathing, a rapid pulse, a loss of appetite and restlessness. Young children who run about in the sunshine are particularly likely to suffer from heat exhaustion.

What can we do about it?

You should make your child lie down quietly in a darkened room, fan him and cover him with clothes soaked in tepid water. He should drink a pint of fruit juice in which a teaspoonful of salt has been dissolved.

When should we call the doctor?

You should call the doctor if your child faints, goes unconscious or does not make a complete recovery within an hour.

Heat stroke

What is it?

Heat stroke is similar to heat exhaustion but rather more dramatic. It occurs after prolonged exposure to heat.

When the external heat is too high the body's temperature-regulating mechanism just cannot cope and the body heats up. The heat stroke victim will be red-faced with hot dry skin and will have a high temperature. The breathing will be noisy, the pulse will be fast and unconsciousness is common. Victims who remain conscious will usually be confused and delirious.

Heat stroke can occur in babies and young children who are wrapped up too warmly and kept close to the fire.

How dangerous is heat stroke?

It is very dangerous and can lead to brain damage and even death. The high temperature can literally cook the brain cells. Convulsions are an early sign that the brain is being damaged.

What can we do about it?

It is important to get the child's temperature down but it is dangerous to do this too quickly. Take off the child's clothes and get him out of the heat but don't try cooling him yourself. Call a doctor immediately.

How can we prevent heat stroke?

To protect your children in unexpected hot weather you should make sure that they become used to the heat slowly. You should keep them in the shade as much as possible, you should provide them with loose, cool clothing and plenty of fluids. Floppy hats are useful and suntan creams will help provide some protection.

Remember that very young children are unlikely to know that they're getting too hot until it is too late.

Hernia

What is it?
A hernia or rupture occurs when tissue normally contained within a body cavity protrudes through a weakness in the muscle wall of the cavity.

There are two particularly common types of hernia in children. Commoner in babies and small children is the umbilical hernia which, as its name suggests, consists of a swelling around the navel. This type of hernia, most common among babies of African origin, becomes more easily visible when the child coughs or cries and can develop into quite a large protrusion.

The other type of hernia common in children is the inguinal hernia which may be present and visible from birth. This type of hernia appears first as a small bulge just above the midpoint of the groin crease. The bulge consists of a sac which contains a small piece of intestine and it may enlarge until it enters the scrotum of a boy or the labia of a girl. Like the umbilical hernia the inguinal hernia is more easily seen when the child coughs or cries because the intra-abdominal pressure rises under those circumstances and the size of the hernia grows accordingly. Inguinal hernias are commoner in boys than girls.

When is a hernia dagerous?
An umbilical hernia is rarely much of a problem. An inguinal hernia can be troublesome because there is a risk that the bowel which is inside the hernia may become trapped. If this happens the blood supply to the bowel will be cut off and the piece of bowel may be destroyed. This is called strangulation and it is particularly likely to happen in babies and young children.

What can we do about an umbilical hernia?
Mothers used to bind their children's umbilical hernias into place in the mistaken belief that this would help them disappear. There also used to be a myth that if you taped a coin over an umbilical hernia it would get better quicker. There is no truth in that myth either.

Umbilical hernias, which seem to affect something like one in every six babies, invariably disappear by themselves by the time a child is 5 years old. Taping something over an umbilical hernia may actually slow down the rate at which it heals.

When do we need to see a doctor about an umbilical hernia?
If your child has an umbilical hernia which doesn't go back with
gentle pressure then you should see a doctor straightaway. If
your child seems to be in pain with an umbilical hernia then a
doctor's advice should be sought. If your child has an umbilical
hernia which lasts after the child reaches the age of 5 then
medical advice should be sought since surgical intervention may
now be required.

What can we do about an inguinal hernia?
An inguinal hernia can usually be pushed back into the
abdominal cavity with a little gentle pressure and by reassuring
the child. A child who is crying or tense will push his hernia out
again as fast as you push it in. There is no point in using a belt or
a truss since this is more likely to do harm than good. Putting a
child in a warm bath may help relax the muscles. If you can't
push an inguinal hernia back out of sight then you need medical
advice straightaway.

When do we need to see a doctor about an inguinal hernia?
You should always seek medical advice if your child has an
inguinal hernia because there is a risk that the hernia will
strangulate or get stuck. If this happens your child will usually be
in a great deal of pain and will also usually vomit. Urgent medical
attention is required and you shouldn't try to push a strangulated
hernia back into the abdomen.

If an inguinal hernia is soft and can be pushed back into the
abdomen you should make an appointment to see your doctor as
soon as is convenient.

What will the doctor do?
He will arrange for your child to be seen by a surgeon. The
surgeon will repair the weakness and since hernias often appear
on both sides may look for a hernia in the other groin as well. If
the hernia is strangulated the operation will be performed without
delay.

Hiccups (also spelt hiccough)

What causes it?

Hiccups are caused by a sudden, intermittent, spasmodic contraction of the diaphragm. They can be annoying and embarrassing but they are not usually dangerous. Nor are they usually indicative of any underlying serious pathology.

Babies hiccup a great deal, probably because the nerve which controls the diaphragm hasn't been properly brought under control. Hiccups are particularly common after feeding. Even in the womb hiccuping is common and many mothers notice their baby moving in the regular pattern of hiccups. This movement is usually fairly easy to distinguish from the less even type of movement that is caused by 'kicking'.

In older children hiccups are also commonest after feeding. they are usually due to eating too much or eating too quickly.

What can we do about it?

There are very many old wives' tales about what to do about hiccups. Some of the remedies seem to work although whether they work or simply happen to coincide with the end of the hiccuping is open to debate!

It is said that frightening the patient helps, that drinking water out of the wrong side of a glass is a cure and that holding the breath will almost certainly work. Sneezing, gargling or tickling the nose are also recommended by some old wives.

Of all the remedies which I've heard about the two that are probably most effective are swallowing a teaspoonful of granulated sugar or breathing in and out of a brown paper bag.

I suspect that the raw sugar may work by scraping against the back of the throat and stimulating a nerve which suppresses the hiccups. Breathing in and out of a paper bag probably works by altering the concentration of carbon dioxide breathed in.

When do we need to see a doctor?

Hiccuping will almost always disappear by itself. You should only get in touch with a doctor if your child's hiccups are proving extremely distressing, are interfering with eating habits or have lasted for more than twenty-four hours.

What will the doctor do?
There are no magical cures but there are one or two rather obscure disorders that can cause hiccuping and there are one or two drugs available only on prescription that may be worth trying.

Hoarseness

What is it?
The child who speaks, whispers or cries in a lower, harsher pitch than usual is hoarse.

What causes it?
Anything which interferes with the way in which the vocal cords vibrate can damage the voice. Mild damage produces mild hoarseness. Severe damage can produce a total loss of speech.

The commonest cause of hoarseness in children is probably shouting and screaming – excited children at parties often have difficulty in communicating the day afterwards. The overenthusiastic use of the voice produces swollen vocal cords and that affects the ease with which the cords vibrate.

If the hoarseness is accompanied by a sore throat, a cough, catarrh, wheezing, fever or the symptoms of a cold then there is, of course, a significant chance that the hoarseness is due to an infection of the nose, chest and throat.

Children who swallow foreign objects or abrasive substances of any kind may suffer afterwards from hoarseness.

If hoarseness is a common, recurrent problem then the child may have acquired some tiny wart-like growths on the vocal cords. These growths usually result from over-use of the vocal cords and are known as 'singer's nodes' in those who follow that profession and 'screamer's nodes' in children who have usually acquired them by the route the name suggests.

What can we do about it?
First, if you suspect that the hoarseness is the result of your child swallowing a foreign object of any kind or drinking any dangerous liquid then you must seek medical advice straightaway.

Next, try and persuade your child to rest his voice. Anyone

who is hoarse and who continues to try and use his voice will make things worse. Give him a notebook and a pencil and tell him that he must write things down if he wants to communicate. You can make it into a game if you like.

Drinking warm liquids helps and the hot lemon drink I describe on page 81 is as good as anything. A steam inhalation is also an excellent way to relieve the symptoms and I describe how to organise one of these on page 81. Holding a hot towel to the neck is a favourite trick that recurs in many old wives' tales and I think you'll find that it may help.

Obviously if the hoarseness is accompanied by any other symptoms then you should also aim to treat those symptoms too.

When should we see the doctor?

If the hoarseness is not accompanied by any other symptoms then it is unlikely to need medical attention. If it persists for more than five days or continues to get worse despite your having tried the treatment methods I've described then you should visit your doctor and obtain his advice.

What will the doctor do?

A family doctor will probably restrict his examination to a study of the throat with the aid of a small torch and a tongue depressor. He won't be able to see the vocal cords. If he thinks the hoarseness merits an examination by a specialist then he will probably arrange a referral to an ear, nose and throat specialist who can study the vocal cords with the aid of special lights and mirrors.

Only very rarely indeed do children need surgery for hoarseness.

Impetigo

What is it?

Impetigo is a highly contagious skin infection which usually starts as a small, fairly innocuous-looking blister. The blister, which contains yellow pus, bursts to leave an open sore that gradually hardens into a yellowed scab. The pus that leaks from the blister spreads over the surrounding skin very easily so impetigo can quickly turn from a small blister into a large patch of crusty, scabby skin.

What causes it?
The organism responsible for the development of impetigo is usually either a streptococcus or a staphylococcus. The infecting organism is easily passed on from one child to another and impetigo travels around schools very easily. Children can acquire impetigo regardless of how careful they and their parents are with their personal hygiene.

How do we make the diagnosis
If your child has an infected patch of skin which is marked with small burst blisters, open sores or yellowish-coloured scabs then he probably has impetigo.

What can we do about it?
1 Although the infected area might look fairly insignificant treat it with respect. Impetigo is very infectious and if ignored may be difficult to eradicate later.

2 Cover the infected area with a dry loose dressing to stop your child scratching it, to prevent the organisms being rubbed on to the surrounding skin and to cut down the risk of the infection being passed on to someone else. If the area is properly covered there is no reason why your child should not go to school.

3 Medical opinion is divided about whether the crusts and scabs of impetigo are best left or removed but if there are only one or two fairly new crusts then you're probably better off removing them with a soft cloth and some soap and water. The organisms which produce impetigo can thrive under the skin and only by removing the scabs will you be able to get at the infection effectively.

4 Keep your child's towel, face cloth and clothes separate from those of other members of the family to prevent the infection spreading. Make sure you wash your hands thoroughly with soap and water after touching the infected area. Adults are not immune to impetigo.

5 Visit your own family doctor as soon as possible to obtain either an antibiotic ointment, a course of antibiotic tablets or a penicillin injection. Your doctor will decide which treatment is most appropriate according to the condition of the skin and, possibly, the results of any culture tests he may arrange.

Indigestion

What is it?

A pain or discomfort which is usually confined to the upper part of the abdomen and the lower part of the chest. It is a very common symptom among adults but relatively rare among children. The pain is often accompanied by nausea, by the production of unusually large amounts of wind, by vomiting and by an unpleasant taste in the mouth.

What causes it?

Under normal circumstances the stomach produces a large amount of acid which is designed to help digest food. If the wrong sorts of food are eaten or foods are eaten at the wrong time or too much acid is produced then the acid may begin to eat away at the stomach lining.

Stress, anxiety and worry are among the commonest causes of indigestion. It is now well recognised that excessive stress increases the rate at which acid is produced in the stomach.

Most of the symptoms which parents ascribe to indigestion are in fact due to wind (see page 251).

What can we do about it?

If a child has an indigestion-type pain on very rare occasions then the pain is probably the result of the child eating too much or eating too quickly. The sort of rich foods that are eaten at Christmas can cause indigestion-type pains in a child. Eating green apples in large quantities can produce an indigestion-type pain. This is probably due to the fact that the sour apples aren't chewed properly but are swallowed in large lumps which are difficult to digest properly.

A small amount of antacid mixture may help relieve the immediate symptoms and it is probably wise to take the opportunity to offer a short talk on the perils of overeating.

If a child has persistent indigestion pains then the chances are high that something is upsetting him. Try and find out what the problem is since the symptoms may otherwise get worse.

It is not unknown for young children to develop peptic ulceration as a result of worry and anxiety.

When do we need to see the doctor?

You should see the doctor about any indigestion-type pains which persist for more than five days or which recur. You should also see the doctor if you are uncertain about the cause of the pains of which your child is complaining or if you are uncertain about the diagnosis.

Infectious mononucleosis

What is it?

A virus disease also known as glandular fever. It is caused by an organism known as the Epstein-Barr virus.

Is it infectious?

Yes. Infectious mononucleosis is transmitted by droplet infections from the nose and throat. It is commonly known as the 'kissing disease' because of the way it is often passed on from one sufferer to the next. This may explain why infectious mononucleosis is relatively uncommon among young children but very common among teenagers.

When will we know if our child has caught infectious mononucleosis?

The incubation period varies from one week to six weeks.

How do we make the diagnosis?

The first symptom is usually a sore throat. This may or may not be accompanied by a red rash, a fever, swollen glands and some abdominal tenderness. These aren't definite symptoms and the diagnosis is usually only suspected when the initial sore throat drags on for longer than might otherwise be suspected and when the patient also complains of a general and persistent feeling of general malaise and weariness.

What can we do about it?

There is no specific home treatment for infectious mononucleosis but there are two things that you should remember.

1 Children with infectious mononucleosis will often remain weak and weary for weeks or even months after the acute stage of the illness is over. During the long convalescence period children

can resume normal activities and return to school as and when they feel able to do so.

2 Children with infectious mononucleosis may also be tearful and depressed for a considerable time after the first symptoms have subsided.

When should we see the doctor?

If your child has a persistent sore throat (I would define a sore throat as persistent if it lasts for more than seven days or isn't showing any signs of improvement after five days) and/or complains of a generalised weakness, then you should see your doctor. You should see your doctor if for any other reason you suspect that your child has infectious mononucleosis since the diagnosis can only be made accurately when blood tests are done.

What will the doctor do?

The first thing he'll do will be to examine your child. He will be looking for enlarged glands and for any signs of an enlarged spleen. The spleen enlarges because it is part of the same system of the body as the lymph glands. Next your doctor will probably arrange for a blood test. There is a specific blood test which will usually confirm the existence of any infectious mononucleosis virus. This test may, however, have to be repeated since it is sometimes negative during the early stages of the illness.

If your child has a persistent sore throat your doctor may also take a throat swab and try to culture any causative organisms.

Some doctors believe that steroid drugs can be used to help children with infectious mononucelosis. This is, however, a contentious point and your doctor may feel that no specific treatment is possible.

Ingrowing toenails

What is it?

This is one condition in which the name really says it all! The redness, pain and perhaps swelling that develops in the tissue alongside the toenail is produced by the fact that the tissue has been pierced by the nail. The big toes are the ones most commonly affected.

What causes it?

Ingrowing toenails develop when the nail has been cut or trimmed in such a way that a sharp edge is left sticking out and is gradually pushed into the skin. When the skin has been broken by the nail it is easy for infective organisms to get into the tissues. Since the nail remains where it is and the skin remains broken there is little chance of the wound healing.

Although this is the commonest scenario it is possible for the nail to pierce the skin and the subsequent infection to develop as a result of a child wearing ill-fitting shoes. An ingrowing toenail can even develop if a child's foot is accidentally stepped on.

How do we make the diagnosis?

If your child has a toe that is swollen, red and painful on one side of the nail then you can make a diagnosis of an ingrowing toenail with some certainty. The infected tissue may become so swollen that it spreads out across the nail itself.

What can wo do about it?

Remove the piece of nail which is growing into the flesh through the skin. The condition cannot possibly heal until the errant toenail corner has been removed. Once the invading nail has been removed the problem will probably clear up by itself although any infection that is present may need to be dealt with by bathing the area with an antiseptic solution. If the infection is so bad that the swelling, tenderness and pain prevents you from reaching the toenail with scissors or clippers then it will help to treat the infection first. You won't be able to eradicate the infection entirely until the nail is removed from the flesh but if you can control the infection you may find it easier to deal with the nail.

How can we stop it happening?

1 Make sure that your child wears shoes that are large enough and which do not compress the toes. See page 286 for advice on buying footwear.
2 When cutting the toenails make sure that they are cut straight across so that the corners of the growing nail cannot grow into the skin. Don't be tempted to cut the toenails too short.

When do we need to see the doctor?
If you cannot remove and cut the ingrowing nail or you cannot clear up the infection within a few days then you must seek medical advice.

What will the doctor do?
He will be able to remove the part of the nail that has grown into the skin after anaesthetising the toe. He will also be able to treat the infection by using an antibiotic cream or antibiotic tablets.

If the nail is too badly deformed to treat the problem by simply attending to the ingrowing portion then a surgeon may have to remove the whole of the toe nail under a general anaesthetic.

Itching

What is it?
An irritating, teasing disorder affecting the skin and best relieved by scratching. The proper medical term is pruritis.

What causes it?
Simple dry skin is the commonest cause of skin irritation in children. Normally skin texture is maintained by the secretions produced by the glands within the skin. These secretions help maintain the elasticity of the skin and help preserve moisture. Some children produce excessive secretions and have rather greasy skin; other children don't produce enough secretions and naturally have rather dry skin. Several things can make this dryness worse. Too much bathing, too much sunshine and too much exposure to strong chemical substances such as detergents can, for example, help make the skin become dry.

There isn't much difference between very dry skin and mild eczema (see page 120) and indeed most children who have eczema or dermatitis of any kind will tend to itch a good deal. As far as the skin is concerned it doesn't make any difference whether the eczema developed naturally or as a result of exposure to some irritant substance.

Allergies of almost all kinds can also cause generalised itching.

Scabies causes a generalised itch because the mite that is responsible for the infection tends to move around the body fairly quickly. Fleas can also cause a fairly widespread type of itch although to begin with they usually cause a localised swelling and itchiness. When chickenpox is the cause of a generalised itch there is usually pretty good evidence of the presence of the disease.

Less commonly conditions which affect the whole body such as diabetes, jaundice and some kidney problems can cause generalised itching.

In many instances itching seems to develop for no very good reason at all, being then made worse when the skin is scratched with the result that a vicious circle is formed.

When itching is confined to one particular part of the body it is usually easier to make a specific diagnosis. Itchy feet are commonly a symptom of athlete's foot. When itching is confined to the anus and is worse at night it is frequently a symptom of worms. When itching is only bad around the eyes it is usually the result of a localised allergy and in young girls the commonest cause is the borrowing of mother's make-up. An itchiness in the vaginal area is usually a symptom of a mild vaginal infection. Psoriasis can cause itchiness which is usually worse at the sites of the disease.

Finally, it shouldn't be forgotten, of course, that woollen clothes often cause itching.

What can we do about it?
Calamine lotion soothes inflamed, irritated and itchy skin and antihistamine tablets will often relieve generalised or localised itching. The best solution is to find the cause and treat that!

When do we need to see the doctor?
If itching persists for more than five days and you are unable to make any firm diagnosis then you should seek medical advice. Your doctor will prescribe treatment appropriate to the cause.

Jaundice

What is it?
Jaundice is a symptom, not a disease. The word simply denotes that the skin is yellow, usually as a result of the deposition of bile pigments in the tissues. These pigments come from the breakdown of old red blood cells and normally the pigments are

turned into bile, carried via the bile ducts into the intestines and
then excreted from the body.

Individuals become jaundiced if red cells are broken down
faster than the liver can cope with the ingredients, if the liver is
for any reason unable to turn the bilirubin into bile or if there is
any obstruction preventing bile from flowing from the liver into
the intestines.

What causes it?

There are three main ways in which jaundice can develop but
there are a great many different disorders and disease processes
which can be directly responsible for the production of this
particular dramatic symptom. The bile duct that carries bile away
from the liver may be blocked by a stone or a cyst or there may
be some congenital fault which affects the clear passage of bile
out of the liver. Some drugs affect the liver's capacity to deal with
bilirubin and blood disorders which result in the unusually rapid
breakdown of red blood cells can produce jaundice. A full
account of all the different causes of jaundice in children would
take up a disproportionate amount of space because a few
disorders are responsible for by far the greatest number of cases
of jaundice.

1 Normal jaundice Before beginning to deal with the diseases
which produce jaundice I must just mention that a very high
proportion of newly born babies (sometimes said to be as high as
60 to 80 per cent) develop 'normal' or physiological jaundice soon
after birth. Premature babies are particularly likely to develop
this type of jaundice since their livers are usually relatively
undeveloped and therefore often incapable of coping with the
bilirubin that has to be broken down. This type of jaundice
usually develops on about the second or third day of life and may
last for about a week or ten days.

2 Rhesus incompatibility Human blood can be divided into
different categories or 'groups' according to the antigens and
antibodies present in the blood cells. There are a number of
different blood groups but the most important ones are part of the
ABO system or the rhesus system.

The rhesus system (which gets its name from the fact that the
system was discovered when some blood cells from a rhesus

monkey were injected into a rabbit) is particularly important because of the problems that can arise if a woman who is rhesus negative carries a baby who is rhesus positive.

(The baby, by the way, acquires his rhesus positive blood from his father. If a rhesus negative woman and a rhesus negative man have children there will be no chance of a rhesus incompatibility.)

The problem of rhesus incompatibility which does occur when a rhesus negative mother carries a rhesus positive child develops because the mother produces her own antibodies against the rhesus positive factor. These antibodies destroy the baby's red blood cells at such a rapid rate that the baby's liver enzymes can't cope and jaundice ensues.

This type of jaundice needs immediate attention because the red cells are destroyed in such huge quantities that the baby may well become severely and dangerously anaemic. There is also the risk that the level of bilirubin in the blood can rise to a dangerously high level.

3 Blood poisoning A severe infection in the blood can cause jaundice by destroying red blood cells and damaging the liver.

4 Breast milk jaundice Breast fed infants occasionally develop jaundice because a substance in the milk prevents the liver from functioning properly. This type of jaundice is only rarely serious enough to merit stopping breast feeding.

5 Hepatitis Hepatitis is a viral infection of the liver which can cause jaundice in children of any age. The jaundice develops because the liver is no longer able to function properly and is not able to produce bile efficiently.

How do we make the diagnosis?
Never try to make your own diagnosis if you think your child is jaundiced. The only important question that you should try to answer concerns the presence or absence of jaundice and not the possible cause.

To look for jaundice examine your child in a natural light (and preferably not in a room which is painted bright yellow). The whites of the eyes usually have a yellow tinge when a child is jaundiced.

When should we see the doctor?

If you think that your child is jaundiced then you should seek medical advice straightaway. Your doctor's first task will be to decide just what has caused your child's jaundice. Only after that decision has been taken will it be possible to decide on the most suitable form of treatment. Rhesus incompatibility, by the way, usually produces jaundice which is visible either at birth or very shortly afterwards. Jaundice which doesn't develop until the baby is three days old is usually (but not always) physiological.

What can we do at home?

There is relatively little that you can do apart from ensure that any change in the depth of any existing jaundice is reported straightaway to your doctor. For general home nursing notes see page 272.

What will the doctor do?

To begin with he will arrange for blood tests which will help him determine the precise cause of the jaundice. These tests will, as the jaundice either improves or deteriorates, enable your doctor to measure what is happening with scientific accuracy.

The treatment he decides on will obviously depend upon the cause. If there is a blockage preventing bile from leaving the liver then some sort of surgical operation may be needed. If there is no open passageway through which bile can pass then one will have to be made.

If the jaundice is caused by some failure within the liver then there are very few things that your doctor can do. If your child has infective hepatitis, for example, the only treatment will consist of rest, plenty of fluids and a completely fat-free diet.

If the jaundice is caused by the fact that blood cells are being broken down too rapidly then the solution will depend upon the cause of the red cell breakdown. In newborn babies, for example, the only answer may be to remove the baby's own blood (which has been badly damaged by the mother's antibodies and which is therefore very rich in bilirubin) with a fresh supply of red cells. The baby is given a temporary supply of rhesus negative blood which will remain in circulation until it is replaced by the baby's own rhesus positive blood as cells die through natural wastage.

Is jaundice infectious?

Jaundice is a symptom and it isn't infectious. If your child has jaundice which is caused by an infection then the infection may be infectious.

How can we prevent our child becoming jaundiced?

A good standard of personal hygiene will minimise the risk of your child catching infective hepatitis (which is transmitted by a virus usually carried out of one individual via the faeces and into another through the hands and mouth).

To minimise the risk of a child acquiring jaundice as a result of rhesus incompatibility all pregnant women should visit their doctor as soon as possible during their pregnancy and should attend surgery or hospital outpatients at regular intervals after that. Women who are rhesus negative will be tested carefully for any signs of incompatibility and if there is a possibility that a baby may be at risk an injection can usually be given which will provide protection. In a relatively small number of cases the baby's blood may need to be exchanged. Firstborn babies are not usually affected since it is only during a second pregnancy that a woman will develop rhesus antibodies. For this purpose a miscarriage or abortion must be counted as a pregnancy.

How dangerous is jaundice?

If the level of bilirubin in the blood is allowed to rise unchecked there may eventually be brain damage. Medical advice should be sought at the first sign of jaundice developing.

Joint pains

What causes them?

There are many different reasons why a child may complain of a pain in a joint. I have listed some of the commonest causes below.

1 Trauma The commonest cause of joint pain is probably a simple accident in which the joint is in some way put under exceptional pressure.

If the ligaments of a joint are torn or stretched there will be pain and swelling. This sort of condition is known as a sprain and the joint most commonly affected is probably the ankle. It is important to make sure that there is no fracture (see page 62).

A joint that has been dislocated will look deformed, be difficult or impossible to move and be very painful.

2 Growing pains See page 200.

3 Rheumatoid arthritis This disease can affect children of any age, may affect just one joint or several joints and usually starts quite suddenly. The name Still's Disease is sometimes used to describe the type of rheumatoid arthritis which affects children. Several theories have been put forward to explain how rheumatoid arthritis develops but none of them have yet been proven.

To begin with the child with rheumatoid arthritis usually has a high temperature. The joint pains may spread from one joint to another, eventually settling down to affect mainly the hands, wrists, elbows, ankles and knees. The neck is also quite commonly affected.

Affected joints are often warm, stiff, painful and swollen and there may be a considerable amount of deformity of the joints.

Rheumatoid arthritis in children usually comes and goes. After the symptoms have been present for some time there will be a remission and then quite suddenly the fever will return, the child will be unhappy and the joints will swell again.

4 Rheumatic fever We still don't know precisely how rheumatic fever develops. It seems to be a reaction within the body to an infection with a particular type of streptococcus. Usually associated with damp conditions and overcrowding, rheumtic fever is nowhere near as common as it used to be. It mainly affects children between the ages of 5 and 15.

Rheumatic fever usually follows a respiratory tract infection, such as an attack of tonsillitis, and begins with joint pains which affect the knees, ankles, elbows and wrists more than any other joints. The main characteristic of rheumatic fever joint pains is that the pain moves from one joint to another, usually staying in each joint for no more than one or two days. A child with rheumatic fever usually looks ill, sweats a good deal and has a high temperature. The joints are often red, swollen and hot and sometimes any movement at all is quite painful. There may also be a skin rash.

The main risk with rheumatic fever is not damage to the joints but damage to the heart valves. There doesn't seem to be any relationship between the severity of joint involvement and the severity of heart involvement.

5 Anaphylactoid purpura (henoch-schönlein purpura) The cause of this condition is as obscure as any of the other forms of arthritis-type conditions. Rare under the age of 2 the disease is accompanied by an itchy rash in which the body is covered with tiny spots which, to start with at least, have a deep red centre and a pinkish outer edge. The spots occur most commonly on the buttocks and the lower back.

The knees and ankles are the joints most commonly affected; there is sometimes abdominal pain and quite often the kidneys are also affected with the result that there may, for example, be blood passed in the urine.

6 Disseminated lupus erythematosus Far more common in girls than in boys this condition begins slowly with a high temperature, joint pains and a very characteristic red rash. This spreads like the wings of a butterfly over the cheeks and the bridge of the nose.

7 Infective arthritis Various types of organism can infect joints. There is usually some swelling, some redness and a good deal of pain or tenderness. There is inevitably a fever as well.

8 Osgood-Schlatter's disease This condition only affects the knees. There is usually a painful and tender swelling about an inch below the knee cap.

9 Others Children with flu and german measles sometimes complain of joint pains. There are in addition a number of relatively rare conditions which produce joint pains.

How do we make the diagnosis?
If your child has joint pains you should not try to make the diagnosis yourself but you should seek medical advice. You should not allow your child to use the affected joint until medical advice has been obtained.

The only exception to this rule is when the joint pain is confined to one specific joint, is a result of an obvious injury, and

is causing only a minimum of inconvenience and pain. Even then
if the swelling and pain are accompanied by heat and redness
then you should obtain medical advice.

How can we treat a mild sprain?
Rest is the single most important factor. It also helps to give the
patient a mild painkiller (such as aspirin or paracetamol) and to
use either heat or cold to ease the pain and relieve the swelling.

What will the doctor do?
If he thinks it likely that the joint pain is the result of an accident
which could have damaged the bones in the joint then he will
arrange for an X-ray.

Treatment for the other causes of joint pain obviously depends
on the diagnosis which is finally made. I have listed below some
of the treatments usually offered for the disorders listed as
causing joint pains.

1 Rheumatoid arthritis Aspirin is the drug most commonly used.
It is usually recommended that children with rheumatoid arthritis
move their joints as much as possible unless movement actually
causes pain in which case they should rest.

2 Rheumatic fever A child with rheumatic fever needs to rest in
bed or at least in a chair from which he cannot escape. It is
important that the joints be relieved of all weight-bearing loads.
Bed rest may need to continue for a month or so. The drug that is
invariably used in the treatment of rheumatic fever is aspirin. The
effect of this drug is so dramatic that it is usually said that if a
good result is not obtained within a very short time then the
diagnosis is the wrong one. To keep the weight of the bedclothes
off the feet and legs a bed cradle should be used. To help relieve
pain in the joints it sometimes helps if the joints are literally
wrapped in cotton wool.

3 Anaphylactic purpura There is no specific treatment although
steroids have sometimes been used with good effect. If there are
kidney complications these obviously need to be treated. There
is no real need to keep the patient in bed when he feels fit
enough to get up.

4 Disseminated lupus erythematosus This condition can sometimes be caused by prescribed drugs. Obviously when a child
has been taking a prescribed drug which could have been
responsible then the drug must be stopped. The only type of
treatment used with any real success has involved the use of
steroid drugs.

5 Infective arthritis It is necessary to treat the condition with an
appropriate antibiotic. If possible any pus which is present
should be removed.

6 Osgood-Schlatter's disease Rest is vital. The knee should not
be bent until the swelling and tenderness have gone.

Knock knees

What is it?
When a child with knock knees is standing up straight the knees
are too close together and there will be a gap between the
ankles.

What causes it?
It is quite normal for a child of 3 or 4 years of age to have knock
knees. Excess weight can make things worse, however, and
although overweight children with knock knees will usually grow
out of the problem by the age of 8 they'll grow out of it quicker if
they lose their excess weight.
    In older children there are some relatively rare orthopaedic
conditions which can produce knock knees.

When do we need to see a doctor?
You should certainly see your doctor if your child is over 8 years
of age and has knock knees. If your child is under 8 he will very
probably grow out of it but you should nevertheless seek medical
advice if the deformity is severe or if it worries you.

What will he do about it?
Probably nothing if your child is under the age of 8. If he is over 8
he may arrange for him to be referred to an orthopaedic surgeon.
In rare cases an operation may be needed to correct the

deformity. More commonly there may be a need for some
alteration to the shoes.

Left-handedness

What causes it?
Many investigators have tried to find out just what makes some
children left-handed but as yet there is still no certain evidence.
At the University of Manchester in England researchers investigating the hypothesis that left-handedness results from problems
occurring at birth found that children born by breech delivery
were more likely to be left-handed than other children and that
babies whose mothers were over the age of 38 and were having
their first baby were also more likely to be left-handed.

Is it inherited?
Yes. However, although there does seem to be a genetic link it is
as yet impossible to forecast which children will be left-handed
and which will not.
   More boys than girls are born left-handed.

Is left-handedness linked to any physical or mental problems?
No. There are all sorts of myths about left-handedness being
linked to speech disorders and other problems but there is
absolutely no evidence to support these myths. Any link between
left-handedness and stuttering which may have existed in the
past was almost certainly a result of the anxiety produced in left-
handed children by parents and teacher anxious to persuade
them to become right-handed.

How do we know if our child is left-handed?
If your child chooses to use his left hand in preference to his right
when picking up toys or playing then the chances are that he is
left-handed. About 11 per cent of boys are left-handed while 7
per cent of girls are left-handed.

Should we try to make our child right-handed?
If your child shows a definite preference for his left hand then
you should let him use that hand. If you try to make him change
then you will produce anxiety, slow down his development and

create a variety of problems. Only if your child seems ambidextrous should you encourage him to use his right hand more than his left.

People who are left-handed sometimes claim that some things are made more difficult for them because they live in a world largely created by and for right-handed people. However, in the world of competitive sport left-handed individuals seem to be extremely successful; possibly because the good left-hander will pose problems that the average right-hander will face only rarely. In top class international tennis, for example, there are far more successful left-handers than statistics would suggest likely.

When do we need the doctor?
There is no need to obtain medical advice for a child who is left-handed.

Measles

What is it?
A very common virus infection which occurs in minor, local epidemics.

How do we make the diagnosis?
Measles begins with the sort of symptoms usually associated with the common cold. A slight temperature, a sniffle and a cough are sometimes associated with some inflammation of the eyes which may look like ordinary conjunctivitis (see page 84). On the third day the rash begins, usually starting on the neck at the back of the head. Small red spots clump together to form red blotches which can be seen all over the body. The measles rash is not itchy and by the time the whole body is covered the child usually seems quite well.

Is it catching
Measles is very infectious. It is spread by touch or breath. After contact with an infected individual a child will take a week to a fortnight to develop symptoms. He can pass the infection on to other children before his own rash develops. Measles sufferers are said to be infectious from seven days after contact until a week after the appearance of the rash.

What can we do about it?

There is no cure for measles but there is a fairly effective vaccine which can be used to provide children with some protection (see page 307). Once a child has got measles tepid sponging may relieve a high temperature (see page 135). If the child complains of sore eyes then draw the curtains to exclude sunlight.

When do we need to see the doctor?

Most children with measles do not need medical attention. If, however, your child develops ear pains, vomits or has a headache then you should get in touch with your doctor. Occasional complications do develop with measles (these include pneumonia, bronchitis and encephalitis) and so any unusual symptoms merit your seeking advice.

Menstrual problems

What are they?

Menstruation is the monthly loss of blood from the uterus which occurs throughout a woman's childbearing years. The onset of menstruation is known as the 'menarche' and the cessation is known as the 'menopause'. Stimulated by female hormones circulating in the body the lining of the uterus is built up each month ready to prepare a fertilised egg. If a fertilised egg arrives in the uterus it will settle and develop on the lining of specially prepared cells. If, however, no fertilised egg appears then the specially prepared cell lining will be broken down. The monthly period consists of a mixture of blood and cells from the womb lining.

All this can begin anywhere between the age of 9 and 17, with the average age for the menarche being about 12. Here are some of the commonest problems which can be associated with menstruation in girls.

1 Delayed menarche Young girls who haven't started their periods despite the fact that most of their friends have started will often worry. However, the 'normal' range for the onset of menstruation is very wide. There is not usually any need for concern unless menstruation has not started by the age of 17 years. At that point medical advice should be sought.

2 Very early menarche Young girls who start their periods before all their friends sometimes worry – particularly if they have not been told what to expect. Embarrassment is the common problem at this age and it can best be avoided by the provision of an explanation about what is happening and good, sensible advice on how to cope.

3 Irregular periods Many girls have one period and then do not have another period for several months. This is quite normal. Once a girl has started having normal regular periods and she misses a monthly bleed then a cause needs to be found. Obviously, the most important reason why periods stop is that a fertilised egg has reached the womb. Parents who do not like to think of their daughter growing up may reject this possibility until the very last possible moment. And daughters who are wracked with guilt may encourage this selective blindness.

Although pregnancy is an important cause of periods being missed it is not the commonest cause. Worry is probably the most important single cause of amenorrhoea (an absence of periods) in young girls but hormonal changes and disturbances can also be responsible. Girls suffering from anorexia nervosa (see page 25) also suffer from amenorrhoea.

4 Painful periods Some back pain and abdominal cramps at the start of a period are common. Medical advice should be sought if these pains are severe. Your doctor can either prescribe simple painkillers or else prescribe a hormone treatment which will probably solve the problem. A low-dose contraceptive pill is the form of treatment most often recommended. When a girl has painful periods she is said to be suffering from dysmenorrhoea.

5 Very heavy periods There are many reasons why a girl should have heavy periods or menorrhagia. Medical advice should be sought since most of the conditions which produce menorrhagia are treatable.

6 Premenstrual tension Young girls are just as prone to premenstrual tension as their mothers and older sisters. Headaches, irritability, swollen legs, abdomen and breasts and depression are among the commoner symptoms associated with premenstrual tension. Although the symptoms may vary from girl to girl there is one crucial diagnostic pointer: premenstrual tension always occurs before a period and at approximately the same time each month in the sufferer's cycle.

There are a number of possible solutions. Occasionally hormonal treatment may eradicate the problems.

What should we tell our daughter about menstruating?
You should explain what menstruating is, that it is an entirely normal phenomenon and its relationship to pregnancy. The girl who is old enough to have periods is old enough to get pregnant and old enough to be told the facts of life! I suspect that the majority of unwanted and unexpected pregnancies occur among girls who know little and understand less about human sexuality.

Although I think it fair to warn a young girl that she may suffer some discomfort and even pain with her periods I think this warning needs to be kept as light and casual as possible. Girls who are frightened by their mothers and who are encouraged to think of menstruation as a fearful business invariably suffer far more than their contemporaries.

Migraine

What is it?
A particularly bad headache usually accompanied by gastro-intestinal symptoms such as nausea and vomiting. Visual disturbances such as flashing lights are fairly common. Victims often have an 'aura' before an attack so that they known an attack is coming. The headache is sometimes confined to one side of the head. It is said that about 2 per cent of the population suffer from migraine.

What causes it?
The cause is still something of a mystery but it seems likely that the blood vessels supplying the brain constrict and then dilate, first reducing and then suddenly increasing the flow of blood to the brain. The initial constriction of the vessels causes the aura and the following dilation produces the pain. The reason why the pain sometimes seems confined to one side of the head is simply that the blood vessels on one side of the head are affected.

All this vascular activity is apparently triggered off by any one of a variety of different factors. Chocolate, cheese, oranges, lemons, shellfish, beans, onions, bananas and fried food have all been accused of causing migraine attacks. Stress and anxiety, flashing lights, overwork, tiredness, pain, depression, noise, glare, strange smells and allergies are also said to be occasionally responsible for migraine attacks in some individuals.

Is it inherited?
Yes.

What can we do about it?
If your child suffers from migraine then the first thing to do is to look for any trigger that may be responsible. Once any responsible triggers have been identified, you must do what you can to ensure that your child is protected from that unwanted stimulus. If the trigger is a particular type of food it is a relatively easy matter to ensure that the separation is total. But if the stimulus or trigger is something less specific and less tangible preventing migraine attacks will not be as easy.

Where migraine attacks cannot be entirely prevented a regular treatment programme will have to be developed and perfected. There are very many different drugs available which are recommended for the prevention and treatment of migraine attacks. Finding the right one for your child is very much a matter of trial and error. Migraine can't be cured or prevented with certainty but its effect and the associated unpleasantness can be minimised with care and foresight.

The simple painkillers, such as aspirin and paracetamol, are often as good as any of the more potent drugs sometimes favoured by doctors. Soluble forms of aspirin, effervescent forms of aspirin and paracetamol elixir are thought by some experts to be just as effective as any other drugs in the treatment of migraine.

In addition to painkillers most migraine sufferers usually benefit if they're allowed to lie quietly in a darkened room since noise and light tend to make things worse.

When should we see the doctor?
If your child has regular headaches which you are satisfied are due to migraine and you are able to deal with them effectively then there is little point in obtaining medical advice. Doctors

cannot cure migraine.

If, however, you are uncertain of the diagnosis then you should certainly seek medical advice. Similarly you should consult your doctor if you are unable to control the pain or if your child seems to be suffering unduly, losing time from school or having attacks with increasing frequency.

What will the doctor do?

In recent years the number of drugs recommended for use in the prevention and treatment of migraine attacks has increased many times. There is today a wide variety of products which are said to be useful in the treatment and prevention of this most annoying disorder. Many of these products work very well on a relatively small number of individuals but do not work anywhere near as effectively on others. Choosing the correct and most suitable drug is, therefore, something of a matter of luck. The only way to increase the odds in your child's favour is to continue visiting the doctor and trying new products.

There are a number of specialists (usually neurologists) and a number of specialist clinics where migraine sufferers are treated.

Motion sickness

What is it?

Although it perhaps most traditionally occurs when travelling by sea motion sickness can also affect travellers on trains, in aeroplanes, in buses and in motor cars. Although the percentage of sea travellers who suffer from motion sickness is high so many more people travel by road than by sea that the number of children who suffer from motion sickness in cars and buses is higher than any other category.

What causes it?

Researchers are still studying the problems of motion sickness. From what we know it seems that the special organs of balance inside the ear have a vital part to play. The physiological pathways are still something of a mystery but it is now recognised that any type of regular movement can cause motion sickness. Motion sickness is, for example, common among children who go on roundabouts and swings at the fairground. A good deal of research has been done into motion sickness since officers leading invading armies usually find it extremely embarrassing to discover that a large proportion of their soldiers are too busy being sick to fight. It isn't much comfort but you may also like to know that astronauts also suffer from motion sickness.

How do we make the diagnosis?

Just because a child vomits in the car or on a train journey it doesn't necessarily mean that the cause is motion sickness. Only when there has been several instances of vomiting being clearly associated with some form of travel can the diagnosis be made with any degree of certainty.

Symptoms usually follow a fairly predictable pattern. Patients usually begin by feeling sweaty, nauseated and generally unwell. Heavy breathing, swallowing, yawning, drowsiness, pallor and vomiting then follow. Headaches and depression are two other common symptoms – though the symptoms are so unpleasant that depression is perhaps almost inevitable.

What can we do about it?

I've lost count of the number of 'cures' for travel sickness that I've come across over the years. Some parents advocate putting a chain on the back of the car. Others recommend putting a piece of brown paper up the back of the child's shirt. And so it goes on.

One of the most convincing pieces of research that I've seen suggests that when the brain is receiving plenty of visual information about what is going on outside it balances that information against the motion and is less likely to become disturbed. It is thought that this is why car drivers, aeroplane pilots and bicycle riders don't suffer from motion sickness.

With this evidence as support I suggest that one of the best ways to avoid motion sickness is to persuade your child to take an active interest in what is going on outside. Trying to read or play a game inside the car won't work because the information won't match the information being received through the organs of balance. Get your child to count lorries, to look for blue cars, to spot policemen, to count sheep, cows or bridges but get him to take an active interest in the outside world. On a boat or ship make sure he can see the sea and in an aeroplane it is probably best to secure a window seat for him.

That isn't all. You can also help by ensuring that your child doesn't have anything too rich, too spicy or too fatty before travelling. And oddly enough it is worth remembering that a snack while travelling seems more likely to abort an attack of motion sickness than to bring one on.

Of the many drugs which are available to help prevent motion sickness I believe that the most effective ones are the antihistamines. These all produce a certain amount of drowsiness but they do seem to have a useful effect in preventing vomiting. Look for a product containing promethazine.

One last point: don't keep asking your child if he feels nauseous!

Do children grow out of motion sickness?
Yes. Most do. The age of 10 seems to be the peak age for trouble.

Do motion sickness sufferers always suffer on all forms of transport?
No. Some children can put up with all sorts of rough weather at sea but will instantly feel ill if they travel by aeroplane.

How common is it?
About one in three of all individuals suffer from motion sickness at one time or another. Of those a third get sick very easily; a third suffer under moderate conditions while the final third only have problems occasionally.

When do we need to see the doctor?
If you're convinced that the child's problem is motion sickness and you've tried antihistamine drugs then I'm afraid there isn't a lot of point in seeking medical advice. Your doctor may be able to suggest a different type of tablet but he's unlikely to have access to any magic cures. You're probably going to have to stock up with strong brown paper bags.

Very occasionally a child will vomit so much that he becomes dehydrated. If vomiting persists then you should seek medical advice if your child seems dehydrated or ill in any other way.

Mouth ulcers

What are they?
Tiny white ulcers are sometimes found under the tongue, on the inner side of the cheeks or on the inner side of the lower lip. These are known as aphthous ulcers. They can be found anywhere in the mouth. They are very small but can be very painful.

What causes them?
No one really knows what causes them but it seems possible that physical trauma can be responsible. Some children get mouth ulcers when under stress.

Are they infectious?
Although there is a suggestion that apthous ulcers are caused by a virus I do not know of any evidence at all to suggest that they are infectious.

What can we do about them?
There is no cure available and whatever you do most aphthous ulcers will last for a week or ten days. There, are, however a number of products which are said to relieve the pain and discomfort. There is no undisputed evidence that any of these work but they may be worth trying.

When do we need to see the doctor?
You need medical advice straight away about any ulcer that bleeds and you need advice about any mouth ulcer which lasts for more than ten days. If you're worried about it, if it is exceptionally painful or if you're not sure that it is an aphthous ulcer than seek medical advice anyway.

Mumps

What is it?
An infectious disease fairly common in children over the age of 5 but relatively uncommon under that age. It is caused by a virus.

How do we make the diagnosis?

The child with mumps may begin by complaining of a headache, a general feeling of not being very well and various aches and pains. There may be a fever as well. Sometimes the first sign is a developing swelling which appears in front of one or both ears in the region of the parotid salivary gland. If one side swells up alone the other side may or may not swell within the next few days. Occasionally the other salivary glands under the chin will also swell. The swelling is usually fairly noticeable but it also makes eating and talking painful.

Is it catching?

Mumps is fairly infectious. The child who has got mumps will be infectious from two days before the swelling develops until the swelling has completely disappeared. Children who have been in contact with sufferers will usually have developed symptoms within three weeks. Adults who haven't had mumps should be kept out of the way since the disease can be particularly painful if the infection attacks the testicles or ovaries.

What can we do about it?

There is no cure for mumps. The pain associated with the swelling can be relieved by using aspirin or paracetamol. These drugs will also help to bring down the child's temperature. Hard, difficult-to-chew foods are particularly likely to cause pain so fluids and softer foods are better. It's important not to stop cleaning the teeth although this will probably have to be done very gently. There is a vaccine available but it isn't very widely used.

When do we need to see the doctor?

The doctor should be informed if the patient complains of pains in the abdomen or testicles or of neck stiffness. The mumps virus can affect the testicles in boys and the ovaries in girls. Very, very occasionally this complication can result in sterility.

Neck stiffness

What causes it?

An injury to the bones of the neck can cause neck stiffness. So can a throat infection which has spread to the glands of the neck. And mild muscle strains or stiffness that result from unusual exercise or sitting in draughts can also cause neck stiffness.

But the most important cause of neck stiffness is meningitis – a condition in which the thin sheath which covers the brain and spinal cord becomes inflamed. In older children and in adults meningitis also causes vomiting and a headache. In smaller children these symptoms may not be clear and neck stiffness may be the only significant symptom of this important condition.

Since meningitis is a potentially fatal disorder which can be treated effectively if diagnosed early I suggest that all cases of neck stiffness should be provisionally diagnosed as meningitis and that medical advice should be sought as soon as possible.

How can we tell if there is any neck stiffness?
If the neck is really stiff there won't be any problem in making the diagnosis. The child won't be able to move his head. He certainly won't be able to put his chin anywhere near his chest.

Milder cases of neck stiffness can be detected by lying the child flat on his back, putting both hands under his head and lifting the head forwards as gently as you can. If there is any resistance you should be able to feel it quite easily.

What causes the neck stiffness in meningitis?
The muscles of the back of the neck go into spasm because of the fact that the meninges are irritated.

If the spinal cord has a meningeal sheath why is only the neck involved?
In fact there will usually be some stiffness of the rest of the spine but the stiffness lower down the back is usually more difficult to demonstrate. Sometimes a child who has neck stiffness will also be unable to touch his knees with his lips. Most normal and healthy children can do this quite easily.

When do we call the doctor?
If the neck stiffness could be caused by meningitis then it is important to get treatment quickly. If the neck stiffness is slight and your child seems well in himself then there is no need for an urgent consultation. You should, however, still seek medical advice.

What will the doctor do?

His first task will be to make a diagnosis. If he suspects that your child has meningitis he will probably decide to send the child to hospital. There a test on the meningeal fluid can be done by putting a needle into the spine and taking out a small sample. This sample will enable the doctors to confirm the diagnosis and select an appropriate antibiotic. Meningitis can be caused by a number of different organisms and different types of organism are, of course, susceptible to different types of antibiotics.

Nightmares

What are they?

Bad dreams, nightmares and night terrors – the names are different but the basic problem is the same. Instead of sleeping restfully and calmly your child experiences fear and terror so real that he is quite likely to wake up terrified and screaming. The nature of the nightmare may be forgotten by the time he's woken up but he may be quite disorientated for several minutes.

What causes them?

Fevers, infectious diseases and certain types of food are all known to cause nightmares. The most common cause is probably stress. A child who is worrying about conflicts at home or at school, worried about his academic prowess or about bullying by other children, may often have nightmares.

In an increasing number of cases young children are having nightmares because of films and television programmes they have watched.

What can we do about them?

The child who is woken by a nightmare will need comforting and will need lots of reassurance. If he has difficulty in getting back to sleep again afterwards (or on subsequent nights) then it might be a good idea to leave a night light switched on in the bedroom. Alternatively leave a landing or hall light on and leave the bedroom door open.

If your child's nightmares seems to have been produced by a specific illness or by a specific television programme then there isn't much need to take other action. If, however, there is no such simple explanation you should ask yourself whether your child could be under stress or pressure (see page 288).

When do we need to see the doctor?

If your child suffers repeatedly from nightmares and you are unable to find any cause or explanation then you should ask your family doctor for assistance. If he is unable to uncover the cause he may arrange for a referral – probably to a child psychiatrist.

Nose bleeds

What causes them?

The two commonest causes of nose bleeds are bumps and nose picking. There are other causes, such as allergies, hay fever, infections and weak blood vessels and in a very small minority of children nose bleeds may be caused by problems with the blood clotting mechanism. But those are the exceptions: bumps and nose picking are the commonest causes.

For some reason that I don't entirely understand boys seem to suffer far more often than girls. Perhaps they have more fights and indulge in more nose picking than girls.

What can we do about them?

The majority of nose bleeds will stop by themselves whatever you do. That's why there are so many beautiful old myths about putting cold keys down the child's back, about pressing on the upper lip and about putting ice on the child's neck. These tricks work for the simple but important reason that the nose bleeding would have stopped anyway.

Having said that it is obviously a good idea to try and stop the nose bleeding as soon as possible and to that end there are some useful tricks that you can try. The best method is to get the child to lean slightly forwards and for you or him to squeeze the bridge of his nose for ten minutes. It's difficult to judge ten minutes without a clock or watch so time it. Get your child to squeeze his own nose because a lot of children get nose bleeds at school and if mum isn't there to help they may panic. If they know what to do themselves then they'll be able to cope very effectively.

If this technique doesn't work and bleeding resumes when the pressure is removed then it may be that a large clot in the nose is stopping the broken blood vessel from healing properly. To get rid of the clot ask your child to blow his nose. Then start again!

It's important to make sure that a child who has just recovered from a nose bleed doesn't blow his nose or pick it for quite a time afterwards. It may help if you put a little petroleum jelly up the nose every morning and evening for a few days. That will help provide some mechanical protection but it will also provide protection against the mucus drying out and making the area more fragile once more.

When do we need to see the doctor?

Most nose bleeds are insignificant. If a bleed doesn't stop in twenty minutes or so then you should seek medical advice. The doctor may choose to pack the nose with a long strip of gauze or he may seal the bleeding vessel with cautery. This simply uses heat to close the vessel completely.

You should also seek medical advice if your child has recurrent nose bleeds, or if the nose bleeds persist on and off for more than five days. And you should also seek the doctors advice if the nose bleed is accompanied or followed by pallor, breathlessness or tiredness.

Finally, if a child has a head injury of any kind that is accompanied by a nose bleed, if you are at all worried or if the nose bleeding is accompanied by headache, vomiting or sleepiness, then you should seek medical advice immediately.

Obesity

What is it?

Although it is fairly easy to decide that a child is overweight it can be difficult to decide just how overweight a child is and just where the greatest amount of excess fat is stored. Traditionally people trying to find out whether or not they weigh too much study weight-height charts but in recent years these have been subjected to a good deal of critical comment. It has been suggested that since the charts in existence were mostly compiled either by or for insurance companies they deal with an exceptional sample of individuals. It is also pointed out that most of the charts in existence were compiled several decades ago and that since then growth patterns have changed fairly considerably. Critics also point out that height-weight charts do not allow for those individuals who are unusually muscular. Those who object to the strict figures offered in traditional height-weight charts sometimes suggest that it is more accurate to assess obesity by measuring the amount of fat on an individual body. This, they say, can be done by measuring the thickness of skin folds.

I have listed below some of the methods now used for measuring overweight children. Any or all of these techniques may be used by your doctor.

1 Inspection This is the cheapest and simplest method of determining whether or not a child is overweight. A child who looks too fat to an experienced observer probably is too fat.

2 Weighing Weight-height and weight-age tables are easy to find. There are some on page 310. Many doctors say that a child who weighs 20 per cent more than the table suggests he should weigh is obese.

3 Skinfold thickness In some clinics doctors and nurses use special measuring calipers to gauge the amount of fat in a child's body. A pinch of skin is taken, usually in the region of the triceps muscle on the upper arm, and the thickness of this 'pinch' measured with the aid of calipers. The measurement is then compared according to standards on pre-printed charts.

4 Other methods Doctors in special paediatric clinics sometimes use other methods to check children's weight. They measure the circumference of the child's upper arm. They may use special laboratory facilities to measure the amount of water and potassium in the body. And they may use a combination of measurements such as weight gain since birth, waist circumference and skinfold measurements.

What causes it?
Children, like adults, become fat because their food intake is greater than their body's requirements. There is no other way to get fat. When the calorie intake exceeds the number of calories being burned up then the extra calories are stored as fat. This method of storing fat is in the body's best interests but in the so-

called developed countries of the world the occasions when food supplies are so low that body fat stores have to be utilised are extremely rare. The individual who has gained excess weight will usually have to make a deliberate attempt at dieting in order to burn up those excess pounds of stored fat.

That is the simple physiological explanation for obesity. There are, of course, a great many reasons why individuals allow their calorie intake to exceed their requirements. I have listed some of these below.

1 The appetite control centre is ignored We all have automatic appetite control centres in our bodies. These control centres are designed to regulate the intake of food. A study published in an American journal showed that when newly weaned infants just a few months old were allowed to choose what they ate from a range of simple, natural foods they automatically selected diets that were just as good in nutritional value as carefully balanced ideal diets worked out by nutritional experts. The infants didn't only choose a perfect diet but they also automatically limited their intake of food. Other studies have supported these observations.

Many parents deliberately overrule their children's appetite control centres. They encourage them to eat whether they are hungry or not. They force them to take food according to the clock rather than their appetite control centre. They encourage their children to clear their plates every time in the mistaken belief that food is always better off inside the body than in the dustbin.

2 The use of bottle feeding instead of breast milk Something like 80 per cent of bottle fed babies gain weight faster than their breast fed contemporaries and breast fed babies are much less likely to become overweight than bottle fed babies. Human breast milk contains its own appetite control trigger. The composition of the milk changes and becomes four to five times richer in fat towards the end of a feed than it was at the beginning. This change in fat content seems to be a reminder designed to nudge the appetite control centre. It is also true, of course, that when a breast fed baby has had enough he stops sucking. The mother doesn't push the last few drops in the container into the baby because she cannot see into the container.

A baby's eating habits are vital because fat babies acquire
more fat cells than slim babies. In the future the baby with extra
fat cells will have more capacity for fat storage and will therefore
find staying slim more difficult.

3 The introduction of solids at too young an age If a baby is
started on solids too soon he will stand a greater chance of
growing into a fat baby (see feeding notes on page 277).

4 An inherited tendency Obesity does tend to run in families and
children who have one or two fat parents are likely to grow up
overweight themselves. One famous study showed that if both
parents are obese then two thirds of children will themselves be
overweight, while if only one parent is fat half the children will be
overweight. Research workers who have studied twins have
shown that children can inherit a tendency to become overweight.

5 The family background and the environment Studies which
have involved adopted children and their parents have shown
that there is also a correlation between children and their parents
even when there is no blood tie. This is usually explained by the
argument that fat parents are more likely to teach their children
bad habits than slim parents. Eating habits are passed on from
one generation to the next.

6 Financial status has an influence on weight Generally speaking
children in poor countries are thinner than children in affluent
countries. However, when studies are made of children living in
the so-called affluent, developed countries it is usually found that
those children whose parents are well off are less likely to
become overweight in later life than those children whose
parents are poor.

7 The type of food a child eats The reason that children from
poorer parents tend to end up fatter is said to be due to the fact
that poorer parents give their children more carbohydrate to eat.
And carbohydrate is, it is said, more fattening.

8 When and how often the child eats The child who eats small,
frequent meals is far less likely to become overweight than the

child who eats large infrequent meals. Nibbling is apparently less harmful than gorging. Children who eat little or no breakfast are more likely to become overweight than children who do eat substantial breakfasts.

9 How much exercise the child takes Children who take little exercise are more likely to get fat. Children who ride in cars and buses rather than walking and who play few sports or games are more likely than their contemporaries to become overweight.

10 Emotional factors It is always difficult to decide just how important emotional factors are in the development of obesity because overweight children almost invariably acquire emotional problems as a result of their obesity! However, children who are exceptionally anxious may seek comfort by overeating.

11 Endocrine imbalances In a very small number of children overweight is the result of some endocrine abnormality. Children whose weight gain is due to a hormone imbalance are usually rather short for their age.

How common is obesity in children?
In one recent survey 70 out of 200 babies were at least 20 per cent overweight by the end of their first year of life. This is an important figure because other studies have shown that about a fifth of fat babies will grow up to be fat children and a high proportion of fat children will grow up to be fat adults.

What about puppy fat?
There is no such thing. Any child who is fat is fat and that is all there is to it.

Surely fat babies are healthier than skinny babies?
It's as bad for a baby to be too fat as it is for it to be too skinny. The myth about bonny bouncing babies seems to have been perpetuated by those kindly folk who judge babies at garden fêtes and who seem to be inclined to offer awards to the most obese babies they can find.

What's wrong with a child being overweight?
The hazards of obesity for children are very much the same as

the hazards of obesity in adults. I have listed below some of the commoner disorders associated with excess weight.

1 A fat baby is likely to find walking difficult. This means that he'll take less exercise as he grows up. The lack of exercise will simply contribute to his excess weight problem.

2 An overweight baby or child is more likely to suffer from colds, coughs and other respiratory tract infections than a slimmer child.

3 A child who is overweight is more likely to suffer from heart trouble in later life. There is also a correlation between overweight and diabetes mellitus.

4 Overweight children are more likely to have orthopaedic problems than children of normal size.

What can we do to prevent our child becoming overweight?
You should try to remember as many of the following points as possible.

1 Breast fed babies are probably less likely to become fat than bottle fed babies.

2 Wait until your baby is four months old before introducing solids.

3 Don't force your child to empty his bottle or clear his plate if he has had enough to eat. And remember to give him slightly less food next time.

4 Don't use food as a punishment or a reward. If you do your child will associate food with emotional as well as physical needs.

5 Make sure your child has a good breakfast but eats as little as possible in the evening when the body's calorie requirements are at their lowest.

6 Encourage your child to eat when he is hungry as far as possible. Do not allow children to read or watch television when they are eating. The child who eats while doing something else will not be aware of his appetite control centre. He'll just keep cramming food into his mouth automatically, regardless of whether or not he is still hungry.

7 Try to keep your child out of the habit of eating lots of sweets. Sweets ruin the teeth and are usually rich in calories. Teach your child to understand which foods are fattening.

8 Encourage your child to take regular exercise. Too many parents insist on carrying their children everywhere by motor car these days.

9 Keep a check on your child's weight and compare it with the chart on page 310. If your child seem to be gaining weight too quickly then try to correct this. It is will be easier to make a modest correction now than to try and deal with a massive weight problem in a year or two's time.

10 If you are overweight then you too should try to control your weight. Your children will find weight control difficult to understand if they see their parents eating anything and everything.

Aren't there risks in controlling our child's food intake in this way?

Some parents worry that if they try to stop their children eating too much they will develop anorexia nervosa. In fact far more children suffer from being overweight than suffer from anorexia nervosa. Parents also sometimes worry that if they control their child's eating habits his growth may be adversely affected. If a child eats sensibly and has a varied diet (see page 277) then there is no risk of any food deficiency developing. There is no need for any child on a good and varied diet to take extra vitamins or minerals.

What can we do if your child has already become overweight?

1 You should encourage your child to look more carefully at his own eating habits. No diet is going to be successful if you don't have your child's co-operation. Point out the advantages of losing weight, prepare a chart and record his weight each week.

2 Don't insist on a rapid weight loss. You're likely to end up with a sickly, depressed and miserable child. If your child loses a pound a week he'll be doing fine. Keep a record of the amount of weight lost and offer as much encouragement as you can.

3 Try to ask yourself why he is overweight. Could there be any psychological problems?

4 Try to cut out unnecessary foods rather than basic foodstuffs. Cutting out sweets, crisps, lollipops and so on won't damage his body at all.

5 Give him slightly less to eat at each mealtime. It is particularly important to ensure that relatively little food is eaten in the evening. Because our bodies burn up few calories during the time when we are asleep most of the food we eat in the evenings ends up stored as fat.

When should we seek medical advice?
If your attempts to help your overweight child lose weight have been unsuccessful then you should ask your doctor for help.

What will the doctor do?
Together with a dietician and possibly the help of a paediatrician your doctor will offer advice according to the nature of your child's problem. If he feels that there could be a hormonal explanation for your child's obesity he will arrange for the necessary tests to be done.

Overactivity (also known as hyperactivity and hyperkinesis)

What is it?
Most parents will complain that their children are occasionally 'overactive' but the child who truly merits this diagnosis will usually be very excitable, almost always disruptive and difficult to control. The truly overactive child will find it difficult to remain quiet and still for more than a few moments at a time. Children with this condition may also be clumsy, they may get angry easily, they may cry a good deal and they may find concentrating (and therefore learning) difficult.

How common is it?
Anything between one child in ten and one in a hundred suffer from hyperactivity.

What causes it?
Researchers are still doing work on this problem but it seems likely that hyperactivity is due to a fault in the development of the part of the brain which is responsible for filtering incoming stimuli. The brain contains a number of these centres and their job is to assess information from the eyes, ears, nose and other sensory organs and to regulate the body's reactions. When the centres aren't properly developed the child's brain is forced to put up with an almost constant barrage of sensory information.

That continuous barrage of information produces hyperactivity.

It has been shown that children with normal brain centres who were never taught to control the input of information or their response to it will suffer from a similar type of problem to that exhibited by children with hyperactivity. The badly behaved child has never been shown how to control his own responses to various stimuli. The hyperactive child may not have the necessary control centres in his brain.

How do we diagnose it?

True hyperactivity is one of the most difficult disorders to diagnose accurately. Some of the children who have symptoms similar to those exhibited by hyperactive children are mentally retarded, others are simply taking after parents who were themselves boisterous, while a number may simply be badly behaved because they have not been properly taught how to behave.

The truly hyperactive child is, however, almost always moving. He cannot sit still to watch the television, to watch a film, to enjoy a party, to read or to play a game. His behaviour will be annoying and disturbing for all those around him but it isn't a result of any mischievousness or bad behaviour. He literally cannot help himself.

If you suspect that you have a hyperactive child you should ask your own family doctor to arrange for expert advice to be obtained. Recognising and dealing with a hyperactive child needs expert help.

It is worth remembering that the truly hyperactive child will have been hyperactive from birth. A child who becomes exceptionally active later in childhood is not truly hyperactive. And a child who is only overactive in some circumstances or with some people does not suffer from true hyperactivity.

What will the doctor do?

The truly hyperactive child will need special teaching and help from a skilled psychologist. He may also need to be given drugs to help control his condition. Some doctors believe that hyperactivity is caused by a food allergy and so those physicians will usually suggest a restricted diet.

Pain

What is it?

Although it never appears so at the time pain is an important defence mechanism designed to protect the body from damage. Put your hand on a piece of hot metal and the pain you feel will automatically lead to your moving before too much damage is done. Sit on a pin and your nerve endings will immediately send information to activate your muscles. You'll get off the pin pretty quickly!

That's a simplistic view, of course. In practice many different pathways exist and many types of pain can occur. There are stabbing pains, throbbing pains, and pains that come in waves. These different varieties of pain are produced by different tissues and organs within the body. The throbbing pain of a migraine headache is usually the result of changes in the pressure inside an artery. The abdominal colicky pain that comes and goes in waves is frequently a result of muscle spasms.

How do we make the diagnosis?

Deciding what disorder is causing a particular pain can be extremely difficult. If nerve pathways within the body become mixed up a disorder in one part of the body may produce an apparent pain in another area. Children, like all other individuals, can suffer pain where there is no cause and fail to recognise pain when a stimulus is present.

You should, therefore, be extremely careful when making a diagnosis about the cause of a pain.

How can we tell if he's putting it on?

Many children will complain of pain when there is no apparent reason for them to be in pain. Children will consciously or unconsciously pretend to have pains in order to benefit in some way; usually from a little extra attention.

Many recurrent pains, particularly those which occur on specific days of the week, are imaginary and require treatment directed at the mind rather than the body. Do remember, however, that even a child who regularly complains of pains which are psychological rather than physical in origin can still have physical problems from time to time. It is very easy to dismiss a child's pains as psychogenic when that child has cried wolf many times in the past but each episode really needs to be treated on its own merits.

So, don't assume that any pain is put on until you have satisfied yourself that there is no physical cause. If you find it difficult to assess the value of a pain you should always seek professional advice. It is safer and wiser to assume that every child's pain is genuine.

What are growing pains?

Children often complain of strange pains in their arms or legs when there is no obvious sign of any abnormality. These pains can occur during the daytime or at night and they can affect boys and girls. They affect something like one in five of all children and seem to be commonest among children aged between 5 and 7 years.

Although they are often called growing pains these pains have nothing at all to do with physical growth. They may be a cry for comfort and love, a result of poor posture, muscle fatigue, food allergies or bone misalignments. The only thing we know for certain is that children who complain of these mysterious pains grow out of them without any treatment being needed. (One word of warning – pains in the arms and legs can be caused by orthopaedic abnormalities, by infections, by circulatory problems and by some blood disorders. Persistent limb pains should not be dismissed as growing pains until a doctor has eliminated other more serious possibilities.)

There is no treatment for growing pains but most children seem to obtain comfort and relief from a warm bath or hot water bottle, a little light massage and aspirin.

What can we do about pains?

First you must decide whether the pain requires medical attention. If you are in any doubt then get in touch with your doctor without delay.

Having given that warning there is a great deal that you can do at home to relieve pain that isn't serious or worrying.

One of the simplest and most effective way to deal with pain is by application of heat. Warmth soothes, distracts and settles the troubled nerves and can be applied either generally through a warm bath or locally with the aid of a hot-water bottle. The most useful drugs in the treatment of pain at home are aspirin and paracetamol. Aspirin is effective as an anti-inflammatory drug and will also help to reduce a fever in addition to having a powerful painkilling effect. Paracetamol is slightly less effective in bringing down temperatures and reducing inflammation but it is an equally effective painkiller. Both these drugs are relatively safe and can be taken in the recommended doses by the majority of children.

When should we see the doctor?
You should seek medical advice if your child has pain which you cannot explain, which persists despite treatment or which recurs.

What will the doctor do?
The doctor's first job will be to make a diagnosis. He will also have access to a wide range of pain-relieving techniques which can be used both to minimise discomfort during the diagnostic period and to aid treatment of whatever underlying condition is discovered.

Pallor

What causes it?
Mothers often worry if they think their children look pale. The general assumption is usually that the child must be anaemic. Although it is a possibility that must be borne in mind that is by no means always the case.

If your child has been out in the cold his superficial blood vessels will have shut down to preserve heat. Consequently he will look pale. A similar result is obtained when a normally pink-looking child is anxious or frightened. The hormones produced by fear close down the superficial blood vessels to increase the supply of blood available for the internal organs and to reduce the possibility of blood loss should there be any superficial injury. So the anxious child looks pale. Finally, some children are just naturally pale. This is usually an inherited trait – the pale child will usually have one or two pale parents!

Having said all that I must admit that pallor can indicate anaemia! Anaemia can result from a loss of blood, from a badly planned diet or because your child is suffering from a debilitating infection.

How can we tell whether pallor is important?

An anaemic child will usually also complain of dizziness, faintness, nausea or breathlessness. He may have a limited appetite, be rather restless and irritable and be particularly susceptible to infection. If your child has any of these additional symptoms then you should ask your doctor to exclude the possibility of your child's pallor being caused by anaemia.

If the pallor is intermittent, and you can relate it to contact with cold air or with times when your child has been particularly anxious, then there is probably no need to worry about it.

If the pallor is persistent, however, and you can find no suitable explanation then you should seek medical advice.

What will the doctor do?

Although the full range of tests he initiates will vary according to the possible causes he is considering your doctor will almost certainly arrange for a simple blood test to be done in order to test your child's blood. This test will measure the amount of haemoglobin in the blood and will provide a simple, definitive answer to the question of whether or not your child is anaemic.

Penile problems

What are they?

1 *It's too small* Mothers often worry that their child has too small a penis. This may be partly due to the fact that their knowledge of the size of the male sexual organ may have been distorted by subjective experience. (Some mothers may only have seen erect male organs!) This worry may be exacerbated by the fact that the deposition of fat in a small boy is usually organised in such a way that the penis tends to look particularly insignificant.

2 *The opening through which urine passes (the urethra) is on the underside of the shaft of the penis* This is a condition known as hypospadias and it needs to be corrected by a small operation.

3 *The foreskin cannot be retracted* The foreskin cannot usually be pulled back in a small child (see circumcision on page 74). This is only very rarely a problem.

4 There are sores and ulcers around the urethra These are normally part of an ammoniacal nappy rash. Your doctor will be able to make a firm diagnosis.

5 It is not accompanied by the appropriate number of testes The testes are formed in the abdomen and they migrate down into the scrotum soon after birth. For the first few years of life they are mobile and may be pulled back up into the abdomen if the weather is cold. They are usually easiest to feel in the scrotum when the temperature is warm – this means that they may best be found when your son is in the bath.

If you have not seen or felt two testes in your son's scrotum by the time he has celebrated his second birthday then you should ask your doctor for advice. He may be able to provide you with reassurance but if he cannot feel two testes he may arrange a referral to a surgeon. He may operate to bring the testicles down and to anchor them in place in the scrotum.

6 There is a large swelling in the scrotum Normally the testes lie in fluid in the scrotum. If there is too much fluid there then your son is said to have a hydrocele. This will often disappear without treatment. If it doesn't go away – or it gets bigger – then ask your doctor for advice. The excess fluid can fairly easily be withdrawn from the sac.

7 It becomes erect very easily The penis is an erectile organ and it may display its capacities without its owner being entirely aware of what is going on. Unless the erection is more or less permanent there is no need to worry about this.

8 There is a discharge Two types of urethral discharge are normal in the male – urine and semen. Any other discharge of any kind may denote an infection and should be seen by a doctor. The emission of semen is a normal phenomenon at puberty and commonly occurs at night. It needs no action and should incur no distress.

9 Masturbation This is a normal phenomenon which may begin in infancy. It needs attention only if it becomes an obsession.

Phobias

What are they?
Fear is a useful and understandable human emotion. It helps to regulate our behaviour so that we limit our exposure to danger. Sometimes, however, very severe and often quite irrational fears develop. These are referred to as phobias and there isn't usually any real sense to them.

The phobic individual is plagued by fears which are quite out of all proportion, which are outside his voluntary control, which are illogical, inexplicable, and often embarrassing. Although he knows that his response is irrational the phobic individual may panic when threatened by his particular bête noir.

What causes them?
Phobias are often caused by something other than the stated fear.

So, for example, a child who is frightened of going to school (and who is therefore said to have a school phobia) may well be frightened of another child or a particular teacher. A child who cannot stand being locked in a room alone (claustrophobia) may be frightened of being left by his parents.

What types of phobias are there?
Acrophobia – a fear of heights
Agoraphobia – a fear of open space
Aichmophobia – fear of sharp objects
Ailurophobia – fear of cats
Algophobia – fear of pain
Anthropophobia – fear of people
Aquaphobia – fear of water
Brantophobia – fear of thunder
Cancerophobia – fear of cancer
Claustrophobia – fear of enclosed spaces
Cynophobia – fear of dogs
Demophobia – fear of crowds
Equinophobia – fear of horses
Herpetophobia – fear of creepy crawlies
Kainophobia – fear of new things
Mysophobia – fear of dirt
Nyctophobia – fear of the dark
Ophidophobia – fear of snakes

Phonophobia – fear of talking loud
Photophobia – fear of light
Pyrophobia – fear of fire
Schoolphobia – fear of going to school
Siderodromophobia – fear of travel
Thanatophobia – fear of death
Xenophobia – fear of strangers
Zoophobia – fear of animals

How do we make the diagnosis?

Before deciding that your child has a phobia you should look for
the following components.

1 The phobic child will show genuine physical signs of anxiety
when exposed to the subject of his phobia. He will breathe faster,
he will sweat, his heart will beat more quickly, he will complain
of symptoms such as 'nausea' and 'butterflies in the stomach'. He
may panic and he may faint.

2 The phobic child will do just about anything to avoid the thing
he fears. He will lie or cheat if necessary.

3 When a child has a phobia his life will be severely disturbed.
He will be quite unable to live a normal life and the lives of his
parents will probably revolve around a need to cope with the
phobia. A severe fear can produce inconvenience. A phobia can
stop a child and his parents from leading a normal life.

What can we do about it?

Once you have decided that your child is suffering from a phobia
then you must try to decide why that particular phobia has
developed. Normally, the best way to do this is to talk gently and
calmly with your child and attempt to uncover the particular
problems which are behind the phobia.

When a child has a specific phobia you may be able to treat
the problem by 'deconditioning' or 'exposure therapy'. If, for
example, your child suffers from a phobia about spiders then you
should encourage him to learn about spiders and to look at
photographs about them. Similarly, if your child suffers from a
fear of thunder you should teach him exactly what thunder is and
how it develops. If you have unearthed a deeper fear then you
should provide comfort, reassurance and practical help. So, for
example, if your child has a school phobia but you find he is terrified

of one particular bully then you may be able to offer both advice and support.

When do we need to see the doctor?
If your child's phobia interferes with his life or your life and you are unable to help then you should seek expert advice. Your doctor may then arrange an expert referral to a psychologist specialising in the treatment of individuals with phobic anxieties.

Puberty

What is it?
Puberty is the time when children turn into young men and young women. It usually begins at the age of about 10 in girls and at the age of about 12 in boys, continuing to the ages of 16 and 18 respectively. The onset of puberty is influenced by many factors including race, genetics and nutrition. These various factors all influence the production of the male and female sex hormones which govern the development of the appropriate physical changes.

What happens in girls?
This programme may begin (and therefore end) earlier or later. On average, however, the sequence of events during puberty is as follows:

Age 10
The breasts begin to develop with the nipples beginning to appear more prominent.
There is a growth spurt. Most girls of this age are taller than boys of the same age.

Age 11
Pubic hair appears.

Age 12
The growth spurt reaches a maxium.
Pubic hair spreads and becomes thicker.
The genitalia develop.

The breasts develop further.
Menstruation starts.

Age 13
Hair appears under the armpits (axillary hair).
The breasts become larger and more obvious.
The body shape changes with the hips becoming larger. The general shape becomes rounder and more traditionally female.

Age 14
A regular menstrual cycle develops.
Breasts reach mature size.
Pubic hair acquires full adult form.

Age 15
The growth rate slows down and growth finally stops.

What happens in boys?
On average the sequence of events is as follows:

Age 12
The testes begin to swell.
The growth spurt starts.
Pubic hair appears for the first time.
The penis becomes larger even when flaccid.

Age 13
The size of the penis continues to grow.
The size of the testes continues to increase.

Age 14
The growth spurt reaches a peak.
Axillary hair develops.
Facial hair develops.

Age 15
The pubic hair reaches adult shape and consistency.
The voice breaks and deepens.
The penis and testes reach adult size; spermatozoa are mature.
Height, weight and strength all increase.

Age 17
Facial and body hair increase.
The rate of growth comes to a halt.

Can puberty arrive too soon?
If puberty begins before the age of 8 in girls or before the age of
10 in boys there may be a hormonal disorder needing attention.
All cases of precocious puberty should be investigated but in
most cases no abnormality will be found and no lasting damage
will ensue.

What if puberty is delayed?
If a girl has not shown any signs of early puberty by the age of 13
or a boy has not shown any signs of early puberty by the age of
15 professional advice should be sought. In most cases no cause
will be found and puberty will eventually arrive. In a few cases
there may be some hormonal problem requiring attention.

What problems can occur during puberty?
1 Skin problems are among the commonest physical disorders.
An increase in the availability of sex hormones is accompanied
by an increase in the amount of sebum being secreted in the
skin. There are also changes in the anatomy of the skin with the
outer horny layer becoming thicker. The skin pores tend to dilate
on the face – particularly on the forehead, nose and chin.
Problems then arise if and when the ducts through which the
sebum travels from the sebaceous glands to the skin's surface
become blocked. Dead skin cells are the commonest cause of a
blockage and sebum collects behind these blockages to form
blackheads. If the trapped sebum becomes infected acne spots
will develop. Apart from the face, the neck, shoulders, chest and
back are also often affected. Since teenagers are usually
extremely conscious of their appearance these acne spots often
cause intense distress. (See also page 19.)
2 Menstrual problems are discussed on page 178.
3 Greasy hair – like greasy skin – is caused by an increased
production of sebum. There is no easy, permanent solution to this
problem, which can only be dealt with by using detergent
shampoos to remove the excess grease.
4 The change in voice which occurs during puberty in boys is
produced by an enlargement of the larynx. When a boy's voice

breaks earlier or later than that of his peers at school he may suffer some embarrassment. The changes in the voice are sometimes clumsy and difficult to control with the result that there may be some strange sounds for a few weeks.

5 Boys sometimes suffer from slightly enlarged painful breasts during puberty (gynaecomastia). This problem will usually resolve itself without any treatment.

6 Boys sometimes also have wet dreams (known technically as nocturnal emission of semen). They should be reassured that this is an entirely normal phenomenon.

7 Anorexia nervosa is discussed on page 25.

8 Breast development which is excessive or unusually early can lead to great embarrassment and distress. Girls whose breasts are unequal in size will often worry a great deal although this is in fact a very common problem. (See page 59.)

9 Puberty is a time of great emotional turmoil for boys and girls. For the first time in their lives both sexes become aware of their own sexuality and of the attractions of the opposite sex. There are new strengths, needs and weaknesses to be explored and tested. When you consider that during the time when this hormonally induced emotional turmoil is at its peak most teenagers are also facing all the social and economic problems associated with 'growing up', and that it is a time when examinations have to be taken and sporting pressures faced, it is perhaps surprising not that there are so many tears during the teenage years but that there are not more.

10 Venereal disease is a relatively common problem among teenagers. In boys the initial symptoms are pain on passing urine, frequency of passing urine, a urethral discharge and sores or ulcers on the penis. In girls the initial symptoms are usually frequency and pain when passing urine but there may well be no symptoms at all. Teenagers should be taught of the dangers of venereal infection whether or not they are known to be sexually active.

11 Pregnancy is a possibility some parents prefer to ignore. Girls who are taught about sex are less likely to have unwanted pregnancies than girls who know nothing.

12 Teenagers who are experimenting with life will often experiment with drugs, alcohol and tobacco. These hazards should never be underestimated.

Rashes

What are they?

Apart from stating the obvious and saying that they are all visible and they all affect the skin it isn't possible to produce a single definition which describes all rashes in any useful way. Some rashes are infectious while others are not. Some rashes are itchy. Some are quite insignificant and will go away by themselves. There are flat rashes, blotchy rashes, spotty rashes, lumpy rashes and blistery rashes. There are infected rashes, allergy rashes and rashes that no one can explain.

What causes rashes?

I've deliberately made my definition vague and rather confusing because I want to make the point that rashes are not easy to diagnose accurately. There are countless possible causes.

What can we do about rashes?

The correct treatment for any particular rash obviously depends upon the cause so if you don't know what has caused the rash then please don't try treating it yourself. I have lost count of the number of babies and young children whose rashes have been made worse either because they have been left too long without treatment or because they have been treated in the wrong way. The majority of rashes, however, can be diagnosed at home and can be cleared up without professional medical help.

The ordinary heat rash is probably the commonest rash to affect babies and young children. Although it usually occurs in warmer weather it can also occur in the cold if the child is overdressed. Heat rashes usually begin on the cheeks, shoulders, skin creases and bottom and consist of tiny, pinhead-sized red spots. Blonde or red-headed children are most likely to suffer. The first thing to do is to cool the sufferer by sponging with tepid water and removing some clothes. It's obviously important to keep the patient cool. It is also useful to sprinkle a little powder on to the rash. Do remember that detergents and bubble baths may make heat rashes worse.

Nappy rashes are pretty common too and there is a good deal that you can do about these. They tend to be red, rough and rather scaly and they're usually confined to the area of skin covered by the nappy. They are sometimes caused by the detergents in which nappies are washed and sometimes produced by contact between the urine and the skin.

Once a nappy rash has developed it is important to expose the rash to the air as much as possible. Do ensure that if washable nappies are used they really are washed very thoroughly and rinsed well. Change nappies frequently and avoid waterproof pants whenever you can. Disposable nappies or nappy liners are expensive but useful, particularly if a rash has already developed. There are a number of special creams and ointments available but zinc and castor oil ointment is probably all that you'll need. Some creams also contain silicone as a protective and although these may help I don't recommend using any of the creams that contain antiseptic. These can produce rashes of their own.

Allergy rashes seem to be getting commoner. The diagnosis isn't difficult to make since on the whole these appear fairly suddenly, are fairly widespread and itch. When a medicine has been taken in the previous two weeks it is worth thinking of that drug as a possible cause. Penicillin is probably the commonest culprit but any medicine is capable of causing an allergy reaction. If you suspect that a rash may be due to a prescribed medicine telephone straightaway for advice. In some circumstances the doctor may consider it more important to continue with the treatment and it can be dangerous to stop medical treatment without obtaining professional advice. To ease the itchiness usually associated with an allergy rash I recommend the use of ordinary calamine lotion. If this doesn't do the trick then antihistamine tablets or medicines can be tried. Antihistamine creams can cause irritation and I don't recommend them. If you get to the stage of thinking of using an antihistamine tablet or medicine to relieve itching then you should seek medical advice.

If you think that the rash may have been produced by something that has been eaten or drunk then it is essential to stop all new foods and drinks that have been taken for the first time in the previous month. Then reintroduce them one by one at weekly intervals. By doing that you should be able to find out what caused the rash.

Differentiating between the rashes produced by the various infectious diseases can be quite tricky. Chickenpox is usually fairly easy to diagnose because although the infection starts with a red blotchy rash the spots quickly become watery blisters. Chickenpox rashes usually itch quite a lot and calamine lotion is still the best treatment available. Measles and german measles are described on pages 177 and 142 respectively.

When do we need to see the doctor?
You need medical advice for any rash that isn't disappearing after five days. If you are worried about it or there are other symptoms then don't wait that long.

Scabies

What is it?
An infectious skin disease caused by a parasitic mite called *sarcoptes scabiei.* Anyone can catch scabies and it is not necessarily a sign of poor personal hygiene.

How do we make the diagnosis?
The main symptom of scabies is the itching which can be very troublesome. When the skin is examined carefully it is usually possible to see a fairly extensive rash made up of lots of blisters. You may also see the small, lined tracks leading from them which show the direction in which the mites have burrowed. The rash may be difficult to make out if the sufferer has been scratching a good deal for the superficial scratch marks made by the fingernails can be quite considerable.

The rash of scabies can appear just about anywhere on the body but it is usually most noticeable on the hands and forearms and around the waist. There is not usually any sign of any rash on the face. The best place to find the small, threadlike, greyish burrows made by the scabies mite is in between the fingers.

The rash, however, is almost incidental. The most significant symptom is the itching. It is usually worse at night. Any severe itch which goes on for weeks or even months should arouse the suspicion that scabies might be responsible.

How is it caught?
Scabies is very infectious and it can either be transmitted directly from one person to another or it can be passed on in infected clothing or bedding. It can live in discarded clothes or bedlinen for up to a week. It is commonly passed on from one individual to another when they are sharing a bed but outbreaks have been

reported in schools, hospitals and institutions of all kinds. The incubation period between initial contact and the development of symptoms is usually six weeks.

How can we treat it?
Your child should be scrubbed thoroughly in a hot bath or shower, using a rough washcloth or a scrubbing brush. After the scrubbing and a good drying the child should be painted with one of the special applications available for this purpose. Most of the available remedies contain gamma benzene hydrochloride or benzyl benzoate. The substance should be kept away from the face and eyes. This application should be left in place for at least a day and every time the child washes his hands a fresh application should be put on.

What happens next varies according to the type of application used but a second application is usually recommended one or more days afterwards.

When one individual in a family has been diagnosed as suffering from scabies all other members of that family should be treated in the same way and all clothing and sheets should be washed thoroughly. It is possible to contract scabies from animals so if there is a family dog who could have acted as a carrier he should be treated according to the vet's instructions.

When do we need to see the doctor?
If after following the instructions given above and given by the manufacturer of whatever product you obtained the rash and itching persists then you should seek medical advice.

If you are not certain that the rash and the itching are caused by scabies then you should seek medical advice.

Sleeplessness

What causes it?
Quite a high proportion of babies and children will wake up during the night. An equally large number will have difficulty in getting to sleep. (Unhappily most parents whose children don't sleep the whole night through only ever seem to meet parents whose children go to sleep the moment their heads hit the pillow!) A certain amount of sleeplessness is normal. It isn't

always necessary to look for a specific cause and it isn't always possible to find a specific cure.

When children do have difficulty in getting to sleep or in staying asleep there is often a very obvious reason. If the television is on too loud or the neighbours regularly make a good deal of noise it will be hardly surprising if the child doesn't get to sleep. The bedroom may be too cold or too hot. Your child may be in pain or he may suffer from breathlessness. He may be wet or he may be hungry. He may not even feel tired – like adults different children need different amounts of sleep.

Those are all problems which are relatively easy to define. But in practice things aren't always quite so straightforward! Some children won't go to sleep unless they've been told a story. Others won't sleep unless they're allowed into bed with their parents. Some young children manage to run the whole family around their own disturbed and eccentric sleeping pattern. This isn't done out of any active malice: it may simply be a result of a child's natural desire for attention.

When there is no obvious reason for a child's inability to get to sleep, or inability to stay asleep, parents will sometimes look for explanations where there are none. It, is, for example, often said that children don't sleep at all when they are teething and that the baby who starts early will be a better sleeper. I know of no evidence to support these theories.

What can we do about it?

If there is some practical cause for your chld's inability to sleep then the solution to the problem will usually be fairly obvious!

In the majority of cases there won't be a simple solution. The only answer then is for the parents to try to train their child to sleep. Going to bed and going to sleep is a habit. Children often get into the wrong habits and insist on being taken into their parents' bed or being played with in the middle of the night. These bad habits are easier to avoid than to deal with effectively. So try not to pay too much attention if your baby starts to cry at night and you're confident that there isn't any serious problem or irritation causing his tears. See that all is well if he cries out but don't keep running into his room if he whimpers. Don't get him out of bed to stop him crying. If you do you'll have found a short-term solution but created a long-term problem. Don't keep going into your child's room to check that all is well because if you do your child will eventually get into the habit of lying awake waiting for your next visit.

The quickest way to deal with a child who won't go off to sleep by himself and who insists on crying for attention every night is, of course, to avoid responding at all for several nights. Most children may cry for an hour or so on the first night but will, by the fourth night, have given up trying.

Most parents find this solution far too drastic and need to do things rather more gently. The slower approach simply involves responding slightly less week by week. For the first week you should respond and sit down on your child's bed. For the second week you should go into your child's room, check that there are no problems, talk to him but don't sit down on his bed. In the third week you should go into his room but don't go any further than the door. And in the fourth week you merely talk through the door.

These solutions will work. Their effectiveness depends on your being anxious to ensure that your child does establish some sort of acceptable sleep pattern.

If you don't really mind getting up every night then you won't succeed in breaking your child of his sleeping pattern.

What about early morning waking?
Occasional early morning waking is normal enough. At special times of the year, Christmas and birthdays for example, it is only natural for a child to wake up and want to look at his presents.

When early morning waking persists around the year it can be quite a nuisance. Make sure that there are plenty of toys and games in your child's room and then hope that he will amuse himself until you're ready to get up.

When do we need to see the doctor?
If you have tried as hard as you can and you still can't manage to get your child to sleep or to break him of the habit of getting up at night and coming into your room then you should ask your doctor for help.

What will the doctor do?
If he is convinced that you've tried everything else he may prescribe a medicine to help drug your child at night.

I do stress that no child should be given a sleeping tablet or medicine regularly. The treatment should only be used for a week. If it hasn't worked at the end of that time then the chances of it working if used for longer are not high.

Sore throat

What causes it?
Most simple, uncomplicated sore throats are caused by viruses or by streptococcal infections.

What's the difference between a sore throat and tonsillitis?
At the back of every child's mouth there are two small lumps of lymph tissue. Known as the tonsils these glands are there to guard the air passageway and to catch any infections which might otherwise penetrate further into the body. At the back of the nasal cavity there is more lymph tissue – this time called the adenoids. And all around the body at strategic spots there are other lymph glands, positioned in such a way as to make them most effective in preventing infective organisms from getting further into the body.

Under normal circumstances the tonsils do a difficult job extremely well. They prevent infections from spreading and they are capable of destroying bacteria which might otherwise have taken infections deep into the body.

Problems arise when the tonsils are so badly infected and so filled with bacteria that their effectiveness as defence mechanisms is destroyed. When that happens, instead of being useful guard posts, the tonsils themselves become sites of infection.

How do we tell what sort of sore throat our child has got?
Differentiating between a viral sore throat and a streptococcal sore throat isn't easy. Nor is it easy to be certain when the tonsils have stopped acting as defensive mechanisms and have themselves become sites of infection with tonsillitis resulting. Throats are sometimes infected by streptococci even when the primary symptoms are caused by a viral infection.

In practice it isn't possible to be certain about the nature of any particular throat infection without doing laboratory tests. This means that it is more important for parents to know when they need medical advice than it is for them to know how to differentiate between viral infections of the throat, streptococcal infections of the throat and tonsillitis.

When do we need medical advice?
Your child needs to be seen by a doctor if:
1 The glands in his neck are swollen or tender.
2 He has a sore throat for two days or more which is still getting worse.
3 He has difficulty in breathing.
4 He has earache.
5 He has a rash that you cannot diagnose yourslf.
6 He vomits, has a stiff neck or doesn't want to get out of bed.

Is a sore throat infectious?
Yes.

What can we do about it?
Gargling with warm salt water or with a glass of water in which an aspirin tablet has been dissolved will relieve discomfort. Aspirin or paracetamol tablets will reduce the pain and fever of a sore throat. Even if eating is difficult it is important to insist that plenty of fluids are taken.

Other symptoms, such as coughing, catarrh and stuffiness should be treated as and when they appear.

Do white spots on the tonsils always mean that they are infected?
No. Tonsils often contain a white or yellow cheesy material whether or not they are infected.

What is a quinsy?
If a large abcess forms behind a tonsil a great deal of pain will be produced. The temperature is also likely to become quite high. The tonsil can swell to an enormous size and may need incising.

What will the doctor do?
Theoretically your doctor should take a swab from your child's throat and try to grow the organisms responsible. Only by identifying the organism is it possible to be certain about what is causing the infection.

In practice it usually takes several days to obtain a report from the laboratory and the majority of doctors and parents want to do something as soon as possible. So instead of just taking a swab your doctor may prescribe an antibiotic – most likely choosing a type of penicillin.

If the sore throats become recurrent or persistent and cause a chronic swelling of the glands in the neck, then your doctor will probably refer your child to an ear, nose and throat surgeon for possible tonsillectomy. This referral is also likely to be made if your child is losing a good deal of time from school, has persistent bad breath or has difficulty in eating or breathing.

Why are doctors so reluctant to remove tonsils?

Twenty or thirty years ago almost all children had their tonsils removed. Today doctors usually do what they can to preserve the tonsils. It is recognised that these glands have an important job to do in protecting the rest of the body against infection. Although it is a relatively simple operation tonsillectomy can produce problems. No operation should be undertaken lightly or even seriously considered unless all the available alternatives have been examined and dismissed.

Why are adenoids often removed with the tonsils?

The adenoids are a collection of lymph tissues in the space at the back of the nose. Like the tonsils, the adenoids are there to catch any infective bacteria which might be breathed in. Like the tonsils the adenoids may enlarge automatically as they do their work.

If the adenoids grow to such an extent that they fill all the available space it will become difficult for your child to breathe through his nose. This will make eating difficult and sleeping noisy. Overlarge adenoids may remain permanently infected with the result that the breath smells and the ears become infected.

Adenoids normally shrink as children get older. If they don't or if they are causing a great deal of trouble it may be wise to remove them surgically. Since if the adenoids are enlarged the chances are high that the tonsils are also enlarged both sets of glands are usually removed at a single operation.

If the tonsils are removed are sore throats less likely?

Removing the tonsils only stops children getting tonsillitis. It won't stop sore throats.

Do children grow out of sore throats?

Yes. Sore throats seem to be relatively rare in children under the age of 2 years and over the age of 10 years. The peak age seems to be between 4 years and 8 years – probably because during that period children are coming into close contact with many other young children for the first time.

Speech problems

What sort of problems can exist?

Some children are slow to learn to speak, others stutter or stammer. The type of problem is obviously related to the cause and will therefore give a clue as to the best possible solution.

What causes speech problems?

Children learn to speak by listening to and imitating those around them. The rate at which they learn to talk depends upon their hearing acuity, their intelligence, their ability to control the muscles involved in speech and the range of sounds to which they are exposed.

The child who is left alone for most of the day and who does not hear many spoken words will be very slow to speak. Similarly the child who has a hearing problem which has not been identified and corrected will be slow to speak. On the other hand the child who is encouraged to speak and who hears a good deal of conversation may learn to speak at an unusually early age.

One of the most serious reasons for a child to be slow to learn to speak is mental retardation. If a child has limited intellectual strength he is going to be slow to talk. It is, however, almost just as common for delayed speech to be a simple genetic trait. The child's parents may themselves have been slow to learn to talk.

Stuttering and stammering are problems which can be a result of the child having difficulty in learning to talk. There are other causes, however, and these problems are discussed on page 221.

How do we make the diagnosis?

A child who is developing normally will babble at six months, will start to use incomprehensible syllables at nine months, will use his first clear words at about 1 year, will start producing short sentences by about eighteen months, will produce better sentences by 2 years and will be able to name some objects by the time he is 3 years old. By 4 or 5, friends and family should understand him and strangers should be able to understand what he says shortly after that. Stuttering is common among children of below 5 years.

A child whose speech development is delayed according to these simple guidelines should be seen by a doctor so that a proper diagnosis can be made.

How can we help?
Don't try forcing your child to speak but talk to him, read to him, check to see that he isn't having difficulty in hearing (see page 103), and describe things to him whenever you pick them up.

If you think that your child's speech is delayed then you should seek medical help without delay so that a proper diagnosis can be made. It is important to identify children who are hard of hearing since if action is taken early the delay in their learning to talk can be minimised.

When should we see the doctor?
You should see the doctor without delay if you feel that your child is having difficulty in using words or if you feel that his ability to speak is limited or delayed.

What will the doctor do?
Your doctor will check to see that there are no physical problems and that the child's mouth and throat are normal. He will check to make sure that the child is hearing normally and he will exclude mental retardation as a contributory cause. If he thinks it necessary he may ask a speech therapist to help your child. Speech therapists do not teach children to talk ahead of time and they do not spend time teaching children how to speak beautifully – they aim at helping children who have difficulty in producing distinct, easily identified sounds.

Squint

What is it?
Normally both eyes move together and look at the same things in the same direction at the same time. When the two eyes do not

operate in this way then the chances are that a child has a squint. Squints are not always apparent all the time. They may only become apparent when the child is looking in one particular direction.

What causes it?
The movement of each eye is controlled by a number of tiny muscles which are attached at one end to the eyeball and at the other end to the socket in which they eye is suspended. When those muscles aren't tuned to perfection the two eyes will not move together. The result is a squint. The precise nature of the squint will depend upon the position and duties of the affected muscle.

Squints can occur at any age but they most commonly become apparent during childhood. Some experts believe that somewhere between 5 per cent and 8 per cent of children have squints.

What can we do about it?
If you think your child has a squint then you should seek medical advice. There are no useful home treatments that I would recommend. If a squint is left untreated a child may lose the sight in one eye.

What will the doctor do?
Squints can often be corrected by using spectacles, eye patches or surgery. Most squints can be effectively corrected. The important thing is to seek advice early.

Stammer

What is it?
The faltering, interrupted speech of someone who stammers or stutters is easily recognised. The two words are usually used as though they were interchangeable but to be accurate there is a minor difference. The stammerer simply speaks with considerable hesitation whereas the stutterer has difficulty in speaking and also tends to repeat the first sound of certain words.

What causes it?

It is entirely normal for a young child to stutter and stammer as he learns to talk. Up to the age of 5 or 6 it is very common for children to have difficulty with some words and to find that their minds work faster than their tongues. Most children grow through this phase.

Some parents believe that stuttering and stammering are caused by tickling while others believe that there is an association between children who learn to walk at a rather late age and children who stutter. I can find no evidence to support these suspicions. Nor are children who are left-handed any more likely than any other children to have speech impediments.

The major cause of stuttering and stammering is undoubtedly anxiety. In parts of the world where children are brought up in a very easy-going atmosphere it is almost unknown for a child to have any speech difficulty of this kind. A number of children who stutter or stammer in their later years do so because their childhood stuttering and stammering was taken far too seriously by their parents.

What can we do about it?

When a child stutters or stammers after the age of 5 it is worth asking for professional medical advice.

Do boys suffer more from stuttering and stammering than girls?

Yes. There is a higher incidence of stuttering and stammering among boys.

Is stuttering or stammering inherited?

No. Stuttering and stammering are not inherited in the same way that red hair or obesity can be inherited. But both these speech disorders do run in families. It may be that parents who stutter or stammer pay too much attention to their own children when they exhibit signs of transient speech impediments.

What will the doctor do?

If your doctor thinks that your child needs help he will almost certainly arrange an appointment with a speech therapist.

Sunburn

What causes it?
Too much sunshine in too short a time is the usual cause.

What is it?
There is no real difference between a burn caused by the sun and a burn of any other type. The skin is red, there may be peeling and there may be blisters.

In what ways does the sun affect the skin?
When white or pink skin is exposed to the sun a number of things happen. Skin cells are injured and they release a special chemical which produces itching and reddening of the skin. Some hours or days later cells deep inside the skin start to release a substance called melanin which slowly migrates to the surface of the skin. Melanin is the pigment which gives the skin its tan and its purpose is to provide protection against further damage. Dark-skinned individuals already have a protective layer of melanin on the outer skin surface and they have to worry far less about the potentially damaging effects of the sun's rays.

Those aren't the only effects the sun has on the skin. There is also a drying effect and the skin becomes thicker and tougher too. Blood vessels dilate as a result of the heat and fluid may leak out into the tissues giving the skin a puffy tight feeling. Blisters and peeling are common *sequelae*.

In the long term these changes can lead to premature ageing, wrinkling and even the development of skin cancer. In the short term these changes can lead to temporary burning of the skin.

Surely sunshine is good for skin?
It is true that sunshine helps the skin to make vitamin D. But your children can obtain vitamin D from foodstuffs. The healthy-looking tan that white children are often anxious to obtain is bad for their skin.

How do we make the diagnosis?
There isn't usually any problem about this. The sunburnt child will usually complain of red, tight skin. He may find it difficult or painful to move. If the burn is bad blisters will be visible.

Are some children more likely to get sunburnt than others?
Fair-haired children or red-headed children are more likely to
burn than children with dark hair.

What can we do to prevent our child being sunburnt?
1 Limit your child's exposure to the sun. Don't let him sit or play
in the sun for more than a few minutes at a time until he has
acquired a slight tan of his own.
2 Make sure that your child is well covered up for the rest of the
time. Arms and legs should be covered with loose fitting cotton
garments. A wide-brimmed floppy hat is probably the best way
to protect the head and neck.
3 Keep your child in the shade at midday. The sun is much more
dangerous at this time of the day than early in the morning or
later in the afternoon.
4 Children can get sunburnt even when playing or swimming. If
your child wants to spend a lot of time in the water it might be a
good idea to give him an old cotton shirt to play in.
5 Sunburn only becomes obvious after an hour or two. Your child
will undoubtedly keep telling you that he still feels fine. His skin
may, nevertheless, still be damaged. Don't allow him to stay out in
the sun unprotected just because he feels all right.
6 Use a sunscreen cream to protect your child's skin. The most
effective sunscreens are those which contain substances such as
zinc oxide. These products do not let any sun through if applied
properly and are most useful for children with very fair, sensitive
skin.

There are some sunscreen creams available which allow your
child to get a tan without burning. These depend for their
effectiveness on the fact that ultraviolet light comes in various
sizes. Short wavelength ultraviolet light tends to produce a lot of
redness but not much tanning while long wavelength ultraviolet
light does the opposite, stimulating the migration of melanin cells
but doing a minimum of damage to the skin.

The ideal sunscreen preparation should screen out some of the
short wavelength ultraviolet rays while letting through the longer
rays. Chemicals which filter out the shorter length rays include
para-aminobenzoic acid and the benzophenone derivatives. Many
products containing these substances provide protection. Some
are waterproof but can still be wiped off. They should, therefore,
be reapplied at regular intervals.

7 A child who lies on a sunbed, before a solarium or under a sun lamp can get burnt in exactly the same way as a child under the sun. The same precautions should be taken.

8 After sunbathing it is sensible to apply a simple, bland, moisturising cream to the skin.

9 Some prescribed medicines and some cosmetics contain substances which can lead to the skin becoming blotchy when exposed to the sun. Don't allow your child to use cosmetics of any kind when playing in the sun or sunbathing. If a child taking prescribed tablets develops blotchiness do not stop the tablets but keep your child out of the sun or use a sun barrier cream.

10 When applying to the skin don't forget the shoulders, shins and the tops of the feet. The skin there is easily burnt but these are spots which are often forgotten.

What can we do about it if our child gets sunburnt?
1 Don't burst blisters.
2 Apply calamine lotion or a thin moisturising cream to the skin. Do this regularly. It will help soothe the burnt areas.
3 Give him plenty of fluids to drink.

When do we need to see the doctor?
You don't normally need to see the doctor about a simple first-degree burn. But if a second-degree burn (i.e. one with blisters) covers more than an inch or two of skin then you should seek medical advice.

You should also see a doctor if your child has a temperature, is drowsy, is confused or seems ill (see heat stroke, page 155).

What will the doctor do?
He will treat the sunburn in the same way that he would treat any other burn (see page 65).

Swallowing difficulty

What causes it?
Any disorder or infection which impedes the smooth passage of food from the mouth to the stomach can produce a swallowing difficulty.

The commonest types of problem are:

1 An infected mouth A child who has a sore mouth, produced by an infection such as thrush, will find chewing and swallowing extremely difficult.

2 An infected throat The commonest cause of difficulty in swallowing is probably a sore throat, produced by an infection. A child with inflamed and swollen tonsils or with an inflammation of the pharynx will find swallowing very painful.

3 A blockage in the gullet Any child who has swallowed a fish bone or chicken bone and whose gullet is wholly or partially blocked will obviously have difficulty in swallowing.

4 A damaged gullet If a child accidentally drinks something that is too hot or which is corrosive then the gullet may be partially or totally occluded by the resulting tissue damage.

How do we make the dignosis?
A child who has difficulty in swallowing will usually be in a considerable amount of pain. Making a specific diagnosis is less important than deciding whether or not urgent medical care is needed.

If the blockage is also impeding the passage of air into the windpipe then emergency action will be needed. See instructions on how to cope with a child who is choking (page 72).

What can we do about it?
When the problem isn't urgent then it is important to have an idea of whether or not the disorder involves a physical obstruction of some kind or an irritating infection. If you think that there is an obstruction, or you think it possible that there could be an obstruction, then you should seek urgent medical attention.

If your child is having difficulty in swallowing because of a mouth or throat infection then you may be able to alleviate the symptoms by providing a simple salt mouthwash or a gargle containing a small quantity of dissolved aspirin. If the symptoms do not disappear or resolve within a few days then medical advice should be sought.

Swollen glands

What are they?

When anyone talks about 'swollen glands' they are usually talking about the lymph glands. These are small specialised clumps of cells sometimes also known as nodes. The function of the nodes is to provide antibodies and to help stop the spread of invading organisms. A gland that is swollen is simply doing its job – producing antibodies and defending the tissues in its area.

What causes them?

Infections which are confined to particular parts of the body will produce swelling of the glands in those parts of the body. If the lymph glands in the armpits are swollen then there may be an infection in the hand, arm or chest. If the lymph glands in the groin are swollen there may be some infection in the foot or leg. The glands in the neck will swell if there is an infection of the throat. If the glands behind the ears are swollen then there may be an ear infection or an infection of the scalp. If the glands under the chin are swollen then there may be an infection affecting one or more teeth.

Infections which affect the whole of the body can make the glands all over the body swell. A child who has a crop of boils or an attack of chickenpox may well have swollen glands in all the areas I've mentioned. In very rare instances leukaemia (see page 263) and other disorders affecting the blood cells can produce swollen glands. Glandular fever (infectious mononucleosis) is one of the commonest causes of generalised swollen glands (see page 163).

How do we make the diagnosis?

Swollen glands are a sign of some underlying problem rather than a disease in themselves. The first priority is to decide precisely what has produced the swelling.

If you decide that glands all over the body are affected then you should look for some general disorder (a generalised infection, for example). If, on the other hand, you can only find one small group of swollen glands localised to one particular part of the body then the chances are that the swelling has been produced by a localised infection.

To find the site of that localised infection you should simply look in the region of the swelling.

When do we need to see the doctor?
You should seek medical advice if:
1 Your child has lymph nodes swollen in several places.
2 Your child has a lymph node that is continuing to grow in size or tenderness or to get redder despite your having started some form of treatment.

Is it ever normal for a child to have swollen lymph nodes?
If your child has small, pea-sized lymph nodes which are not red or painful then they are probably quite normal. Lymph nodes which have swollen as a result of an infection may take some weeks or even months to go back to their normal size.

Are swollen lymph nodes infectious?
Lymph nodes themselves are not infectious but the underlying, responsible disease may be contagious.

What can we do at home?
There is no treatment that you can provide at home for swollen lymph nodes. You may be able to relieve mild pain and discomfort with aspirin, paracetamol and heat.

What will the doctor do?
He'll want to find out what has caused the lymph nodes to swell. After examining your child he may decide to take blood tests and to send these to the laboratory. The blood tests will tell him whether there is any obvious sign of infection in the blood. They will also provide him with a report on the condition of the blood cells themselves.

If your doctor feels that an infection is responsible and that treatment with an antibiotic will help he will provide the appropriate prescription. If he is still uncertain as to the cause of the swelling he may arrange for the gland (or part of it) to be removed and examined under a microscope. If the gland is very badly swollen he may decide that it needs to be cut open and drained.

Teething

What is it?

Unless they are present at birth the twenty milk teeth which a
child has must erupt through the gums at some time during a
baby's first two or three years of life. This process is known as
'teething'. Teething is not a disease and it produces nothing more
than teeth.

How can we tell that our baby is teething?

As teeth force their way through the gums they sometimes
produce a little pain. There is usually also some redness and
swelling of the gums and there may, in addition, be a slight fever.
The discomfort and soreness may occasionally interfere with
sleep and may make eating some foods rather difficult but
teething is not accompanied by any other symptoms of real
significance. Teething starts at about six months of age and
continues until the baby is thirty months old. Usually, but not
always, it is the lower, central teeth which arrive first (see page
312).

What can we do about it?

Dealing with the minor discomforts which are genuinely associated with teething is a relatively simple matter. The soreness and
pain can be temporarily relieved by the use of an anaesthetic gel
designed to be rubbed on to the gums but such products are of
limited value since they are quickly washed away. Since teething
is a process which continues on and off for many months a
product which provides such a short-lasting effect is not much
use. Children sometimes develop allergies to the substances
included in some teething gels.

As an occasional short-term solution I suggest using either
junior aspirin tablets of the soluble variety or paracetamol
medicine. However, teething pains are not usually severe enough
to merit a painkiller and if a child is in constant or recurring pain
then he needs medical attention.

Biting on something hard often helps to relieve the discomfort
and may even encourage teeth to erupt. This is why so many
teething children suck their thumbs or bite their fingers. A piece
of hard food will sometimes do although special teething rings
are available. Incidentally, biting on something cold helps to

numb the gums and relieve pain as well so its worth putting the
teething ring in the fridge.

Try and ignore the many myths about teething which seem to
be handed on from one generation to another. One popular myth
is that teething causes skin problems. There is no truth in this
rumour apart from the fact that the dribbling which is sometimes
associated with teething may cause a soreness and redness on
the cheeks. To prevent this happening it is usually enough to
apply a barrier cream to the cheeks. In fact the dribbling that
may accompany teething is probably an independent problem
caused by the salivary glands starting to work properly at
roughly the same sort of age that the teeth start to erupt.

It is also said that teething causes irritability. To a certain
extent this may be true. But the other causes of irritability in a
child are so common that it is wrong to blame teething all the
time. The irritable child is more likely to be tired or overexcited
than simply teething. Whatever the cause of the irritability if the
child cannot be distracted or soothed with a toy or a cuddle then
it is probably wise to ask for expert help.

Teething has also been blamed for just about every childhood
condition from asthma to worms, including fevers, diarrhoea,
bronchitis and fits. There are dozens of different tablets,
powders, gels, powders, creams and mixtures offered to help
parents cope with these imaginary connections. Teething is a
perfectly normal process and one which causes remarkably little
trouble when it is repeated later in childhood as the permanent
teeth come through. There is no need for you to do anything
other than follow the simple advice I have given.

Do not be tempted to try the old wives' tale and cut the gum
above an erupting tooth with a spoon or a knife. This is
unnecessary and likely to cause more pain than it relieves.

When do we need to call the doctor?
There is no need to call the doctor or seek medical advice for
teething unless your child is clearly in pain. If that is the case then
there is a very good chance that the problem isn't teething at all.

Tics and spasms
What are they?
Tics are fast, unexpected, repetitive, jerky, spasmodic move-

ments which serve no purpose and which are entirely involuntary. Tics commonly involve the small muscles of the face and may result in winking, blinking, twitching the mouth and wrinkling the forehead. Other tics involve larger muscles and may result in repetitive coughing, sighing, sniffing, flicking back of the hair, shrugging of the shoulders, and indeed just about anything else that muscles can do.

What causes them?

Most tics are a result of stress, anxiety or tension. Boredom can produce tics in a very small child as can insecurity.

How do we make the diagnosis:

Tics are not usually difficult to diagnose but confusion can sometimes arise because some repetitive movements can be produced by allergies, infections and irritations of one sort or another. For example, a child with hay fever will often twitch his nose or blink his eyes in such a way as to suggest that he has acquired a tic or habit spasm. Children with catarrh often develop ticklish coughs which may be impossible to differentiate from a coughing habit.

What can we do about them?

Try and ignore them. Tics and habit spasms are extremely annoying but if you reprimand your child I'm afraid the chances are high that the tic will just go on for longer. Anxiety produces and reinforces tics.

There are no medicines which will help make tics disappear but most go away by themselves as mysteriously as they arrived. If you can find any stresses or strains which are likely to be worrying your child then it will help to deal with them. Try and persuade your child's friends and relatives to join with you in ignoring the problem. About one in five children has a tic at one time or another. Tics rarely last for more than a month or two.

When do we need to see a doctor?

If your child's tic does not disappear after a week or two then you should seek medical advice. Your doctor will be able to eliminate any chance that the tic could be caused by a disease. He will be able to help you decide how best to deal with any stresses which may be causing the tic.

Should your child's tic develop into a violent twitching of other parts of his body then you should seek medical advice. This is also true if you notice that the muscular movement is accompanied by any talking or shouting. In a relatively uncommon condition known as Gilles de la Tourette's disease children have a good many muscular tics but also have a tendency to shout out loud. They may grunt, snort, bark or swear and for some reason the child with this condition will often shout out obscenities or other entirely unsuitable phrases.

What will the doctor do?
If the doctor decides that your child has a simple tic or habit spasm he is unlikely to be able to provide any positive treatment. If he makes a diagnosis of Gilles de la Tourette's disease he may ask a neurologist for advice and he may offer drug treatment. Haloperidol is one of the drugs most commonly selected.

Tiredness

What causes it?
There are times when perfectly healthy and fit children will complain or show symptoms of tiredness. A child who has been up late the previous night or who has been on a very long walk may either complain directly of tiredness or may appear irritable and sleepy. That sort of tiredness is nothing to worry about!

Much more likely to produce concern is the sort of tiredness which either continues for day after day or which recurs. That sort of tiredness does need to be taken seriously. Anaemia is probably one of the commonest causes of tiredness – itself often being a result of a poor appetite or inadequate eating habits – but other causes include an inability to sleep properly and too much stress or pressure. A child who has recently had an infectious disease may be tired for several weeks afterwards.

How do we make the diagnosis?
If your child is permanently tired or repeatedly suffers from tiredness then you should ask yourself three questions:
1 Is he eating well enough? If he isn't then what can you do to remedy the matter?
2 Is he sleeping well enough? If he isn't then there must be a

reason. If you can't deal with the sleeplessness then you must get medical help.

3 Has he recently suffered from an infection or illness of any kind? If the answer to this last question is yes then that may well explain the tiredness. However, the symptoms should slowly but steadily disappear as the days and weeks go by.

What can we do about it?

If you have made a specific diagnosis and you know why your child is tired then you can treat that specific diagnosis. (See page 277 if your child's problem involves his eating habits, and page 213 if he does not sleep properly.)

If you have not made a specific diagnosis then you should not try treating your child yourself but should visit your doctor. Do not buy any over-the-counter tonic or iron remedy. If your child needs specific treatments (for example for iron deficiency anaemia) then blood tests should be done before the treatment is initiated. The tests should be repeated after the conclusion of the treatment in order to determine the relevance and effectiveness of the treatment.

What will the doctor do?

He'll probably want to use laboratory tests to find out why your child is tired. He will then provide the appropriate form of treatment.

Tongue tie

What is it?

The underside of the tongue is normally attached to the floor of the mouth by a small piece of tissue called the frenulum. If you lift your tongue and look into the mirror you'll see it quite clearly in the middle of the tongue's underside.

Very occasionally the frenulum is so abnormally thick and short that it holds the tongue back, restricting forward movement.

How do we make the diagnosis?

If your child seems to have difficulty in pushing out his tongue, try and look on the underside at the frenulum. Then compare what you see with the frenulum on your own tongue or on the tongue of other children. Remember that there are many variations within the normal range.

Is tongue tie a dangerous or incapacitating condition?
It used to be thought that children who were tongue-tied would suffer from speech disorders and feeding problems. (The phrase 'he's tongue-tied' has even become part of the English language.) More recent research has, however, confirmed that there is little risk that a child with a short frenulum will suffer from anything other than perhaps an inability to push out his tongue quite as far as other children.

What can we do about it?
Nothing. Do not try cutting the frenulum under any circumstances.

When do we need the doctor?
If you are worried about the effect your child's shortened frenulum is having then visit your doctor for advice.

What will the doctor do?
Doctors used to recommend that short frenulums be cut. Today most doctors believe that the risks involved in cutting the frenulum (the risks include infection, haemorrhage and the formation of scar tissue which may itself produce more problems) are greater than the advantages. Children can eat and talk quite comfortably without any surgical intervention.

Very rarely, if the frenulum is so short that the tongue is pulled into a concave cup shape, then the operation may be considered. If the operation is considered necessary it should be done by a plastic surgeon or a specialist in paediatric surgery and not by a family doctor or in a casualty department.

Toothache

What causes it?
Each tooth has a root which is attached to the bone beneath by fibrous bands called peridontal ligaments, a crown which is the piece of the tooth which is in view in the mouth, and a neck which connects the two. The crown of every tooth is covered with an outer layer of enamel, the hardest material in the body.

Underneath the enamel is a substance called dentine which is not quite so hard but which is similar in composition to bone. Inside the dentine is the pulp which provides the tooth with nourishment from blood vessels and which is equipped with a nerve.

Pains in or around a tooth can be caused by an infection or abscesses in and around the tooth, by decay which has destroyed the enamel and dentine and exposed the inner pulp, or by injury to the tooth.

However, pains which appear to be caused by bad teeth can be caused by problems in other parts of the face and head. Earache and sinusitis, for example, are two common disorders which mimic toothache in children.

How do we make the diagnosis?
It can be extremely difficult to differentiate between earache and toothache but one useful pointer is the child's temperature. A child with toothache will not usually have a fever whereas a child with earache often will have. If the gum is infected it may be red and swollen. A gentle tap on an infected tooth will produce extra pain and a firm diagnosis.

Making the diagnosis is not so important as deciding whether medical attention is needed straightaway. If you can relieve the pain yourself then you can wait twelve hours before seeking professional help. If at the end of that time the pain still needs attention then you should visit the doctor if you are uncertain as to the source of the pain or the dentist if you are convinced that the problem is caused by toothache. If you cannot relieve the pain at home then you should call for professional help immediately.

What can we do to relieve the pain?
1 The good old fashioned hot-water bottle is probably the best remedy for face pains of all kinds. Wrap a hot-water bottle in a thin towel so that it doesn't burn the skin and give it to your child to hold against the most painful spot. If you haven't got a hot-water bottle then use a warm face cloth or towel. If heat doesn't help then try an ice pack.
2 Give aspirin or paracetamol according to the manufacturer's instructions.
3 Oil of cloves will relieve pain quite dramatically if dabbed directly on to a damaged tooth.
4 Bathing an affected tooth with a little whisky usually helps. You

don't need much and it doesn't matter whether you use blended or malt, Scotch or Irish.

What about 'sensitive' teeth?
The only part of a tooth which can transmit pain is the pulp. Normally the dentine and enamel protect the pulp from external threats of all kinds but occasionally children complain that their teeth are particularly sensitive to very hot, very cold or very sweet foods. This condition can be produced and exacerbated by too much harsh brushing with an abrasive toothpaste. It can often be relieved by the use of special toothpaste containing strontium.

How do we stop toothache developing?
Dentists remove many tons of decayed teeth every year. Dental decay is said to be one of the commonest diseases in the western world. In one recent survey it was found that two thirds of school-age children had decayed teeth and that nearly a third of all adults had lost all of their teeth. Toothache is an inevitable consequence when teeth are allowed to go bad.

To avoid tooth decay in your children teach them how to look after their teeth properly. I have included full advice on page 283. In addition to ensuring that good dental hygiene is carried out you should learn to be aware of the early signs of dental trouble. These are:

1 Bleeding gums.
2 Persistent bad breath.
3 Swollen gums.
4 Loose teeth.

Vaginal discharge

What causes it?
It is not uncommon for young girls to have a vaginal discharge. Newborn baby girls, only a few days old, may have a vaginal discharge of clear mucus as a result of female sex hormones still circulating in their blood. This type of discharge is invariably clear and does not usually smell unpleasant or cause any discolouration.

A similar type of discharge often precedes the onset of

menstruation. Once again this discharge is produced by a rise in circulating female hormones. This time the hormones are produced within the girl's own body instead of being second-hand.

More worrying to young girls and their mothers are the types of vaginal discharge which smell nasty and cause irritation and itching. These types of offensive discharge can be produced in many ways. First, however, make sure that no foreign bodies have been pushed into the vagina. Young girls will often experiment by pushing small objects into themselves. There is no real danger in this unless the object they choose is forgotten.

Many different organisms can infect this area too and a persistent, offensive discharge of any kind needs to be investigated properly if a cause is going to be found. Young girls may also develop a vaginal discharge as a result of using chemical bubble baths and vaginal deodorants or wearing panties made of synthetic materials.

So far I've dealt only with girls suffering from vaginal discharges consisting of clear or discoloured mucus. Vaginal bleeding is also a type of vaginal discharge.

Vaginal bleeding most commonly occurs among young girls who have reached the menarche. There is no fixed age at which a girl should begin to have her periods but the majority of girls start between the ages of 9 and 16 (see page 178). It is usually fairly clear that a girl is starting her periods if she has a vaginal bleed because there will probably also be some breast development.

There are, of course, other causes of vaginal bleeding which need to be remembered. Young female babies of one or two weeks of age may lose a little blood from their vaginas as a result of those circulating maternal hormones and occasionally girls will have some vaginal bleeding after injury because of inflammation or as a result of some sort of growth.

How do we make the diagnosis?

If the discharge is bloody, occurs during the baby's first week or two of life and then stops it is probably due to circulating female hormones. If the discharge is bloody and occurs at the sort of time that a girl might be expected to start menstruating then that is probably the cause – particularly if the bleeding has been preceded by some mucus discharge and some breast development. If, however, there is any uncertainty about the diagnosis or the bleeding continues for more than five days then medical advice should be sought.

If the discharge consists of a clear mucus and is not accompanied by any unpleasant smell or by any irritation then there is no need to worry. This type of discharge is quite normal. If, however, the discharge is accompanied by an unpleasant smell, any irritation or any other unpleasant symptoms then medical advice must be sought.

How can we prevent vaginal problems?

1 Don't let your daughter use any vaginal spray, deodorant or medicated wipe.
2 Don't let your daughter use any bubble bath or put any other chemicals into her bath water.
3 Buy cotton underpants.
4 Tell your daughter to wipe herself from front to back when she has been to the lavatory. This helps to prevent urinary tract infections as well as vaginal infections.

What can we do about them?

Nothing. If the discharge is clear and inoffensive there is no need for any treatment. If the discharge is pussy and offensive then your doctor must make an accurate diagnosis before initiating treatment.

Minor wounds and lacerations around the vaginal area will heal without any form of treatment. More serious injuries need medical attention.

When should we see the doctor?

1 You should seek medical advice if the bleeding is unexplained or continuous for more than five days.
2 Any irritation, any offensive discharge and any itching merits a visit to the doctor.
3 Any girl whose mother took a drug called diethylstilboestrol during pregnancy should see a doctor if she develops any vaginal discharge. Diethylstilboestrol is now known to be a possible cause of a vaginal deformity.

What will the doctor do?

If he suspects an infection the doctor will take a swab. Only if he considers it clinically necessary will the doctor make an internal examination. Most minor conditions can be cleared up without a vaginal examination. A urine test may be done to exclude a urine infection.

Vomiting

What is it?
According to my dictionary vomiting is the 'forcible ejection of the stomach contents through the mouth'. I think that's pretty succinct.

What causes it?
There are many possible causes. Before going on to discuss the more important causes of true vomiting, however, I want to make it clear that regurgitation and the dribbling of fluids and food is not true vomiting. It is common enough for babies and young children to be rather messy eaters. The key word in the definition of vomiting that I've already given is perhaps 'forcible'. If your child is vomiting then the material he brings up will at the very least clear his chin.

The different causes of vomiting vary with age. So I'll start with an account of the causes of vomiting among babies and infants. The commonest problem is simple spitting up of food. The baby who does this won't look ill, won't have a fever, won't have any diarrhoea and won't need any treatment. It is quite normal for infants to get rid of a certain amount of their food this way and apart from being rather messy it certainly isn't anything to worry about. Overfeeding a baby or not giving him enough time to breathe are other common causes of occasional spitting, spluttering and vomiting.

The most serious causes of vomiting among babies will all interfere with weight gain. If your baby is vomiting so much that he isn't putting on weight then you should begin to consider the possibility that there may be something more important going on.

Your baby may not be able to tolerate his food or milk preparation or there may be some obstruction stopping food from getting into the stomach. The most important type of obstruction in young children is caused by pyloric stenosis. Babies who have this problem will usually vomit quite violently, with food being fired several feet at a time. Pyloric stenosis is inherited, the symptoms usually start in the second or third week of life and it is much commoner in boys than in girls. About three in every 1000 babies born have pyloric stenosis and one theory about the delay which occurs between the baby being born and the symptoms developing is that it is the onset of feeding that causes the swelling of the part of the stomach known as the pylorus. This swelling prevents food from travelling on down the intestinal tract and it causes vomiting which can be quite sensational in its extent.

The child who is developing pyloric stenosis will usually begin by vomiting only occasionally. Within a few days, however, he will be vomiting after very feed. And unlike babies with other types of vomiting babies with pyloric stenosis will usually continue to feed quite voraciously. The only solution is an operation to repair the fault. This is usually quite successful.

Coughs and colds and infectious diseases of all kinds can cause vomiting in children of most ages. With babies and younger children the vomiting is sometimes caused by the child's inability to cough up and spit out phlegm. The phlegm is swallowed, it accumulates in the stomach and the child vomits. Vomiting is particularly common with whooping cough which is described on page 249.

Infections of the gastro-intestinal system can also cause vomiting. When they do there is quite commonly some diarrhoea as well. In disorders such as food poisoning, for example, the gastrointestinal system is simply doing everything it can to get rid of the organisms which have caused the infection. The vomiting usually starts first and then, as the bug moves down the intestinal tract, the diarrhoea follows.

Those are just some of the many possible causes of vomiting in children. I should perhaps also mention that children with meningitis will frequently vomit, as will children with appendicitis, migraine and some heart disorders. Children often vomit when they are nervous or excited, they vomit because of motion sickness and they may vomit if they have swallowed poisons or drugs.

How do we make the diagnosis?
Sometimes the diagnosis is fairly obvious. If everyone in the family suddenly starts to vomit after a meal out at a restaurant then the chances are, I'm afraid, that you've all picked up some

sort of food poisoning bug. If your child only vomits when travelling by car then there is a pretty good chance that he suffers from motion sickness.

But making the diagnosis is by no means always as easy as that. And I don't think that it is as important for parents to be able to differentiate between the various causes of vomiting as it is for them to be able to decide when they need professional help and when they can safely deal with their vomiting child themselves.

When do we need medical advice?

1 If your child looks ill. Or if you suspect that he might have taken an overdose or drugs or poison.

2 If your child is complaining of pain (unless you are satisfied that your child has a recurrence of a problem such as migraine which you are happy to treat at home).

3 If you think your child is getting dehydrated. If, when you pick up a pinch of skin, the fold stays clearly visible for a second or so after you have let go, then your child may be dehydrated.

4 If your child has any additional symptoms such as fever or diarrhoea and you are either uncertain about the diagnosis or uncertain about the most suitable form of treatment.

5 If he has had a recent head injury.

6 If your child is vomiting with great force or if he has been vomiting for more than twenty-four hours.

7 If there has been any accompanying weight loss or a lack of an expected weight gain.

8 If your child is vomiting and won't take any fluids.

What can we do at home?

You should not give him anything to eat since food will only make things worse but you should give him regular sips of fluid. Your child can survive happily for a day or two without food but fluid shortage can cause real problems. You can give him what he will happily swallow and keep down. Cool, clear fluids are usually most acceptable.

What will the doctor do?

He'll decide what is causing the vomiting. A minority of children (those with pyloric stenosis or appendicitis for example) will need to be admitted to hospital. The majority can be looked after at home and may not even need any treatment.

Walking difficulties

What causes them?

If you hold a young baby upright with the soles of his feet on a flat surface and you then slowly move him forwards the baby will automatically make a walking movement. He will be responding to an inner reflex. During the years which follow many things can go wrong and children can develop walking difficulties for a great variety of different reasons.

What types of walking difficulty are there?

1 Learning to walk rather late Many parents worry if their child isn't walking by himself by the time he is a year old. They believe that there is a correlation between the age at which a child starts to walk and his intelligence. Some will have heard the old myth that a child who learns to walk late will stutter when he learns to talk. In fact the normal age for a child to learn to walk can vary from eight months of age to eighteen months. And if a child learns to walk between eight and eighteen months there is absolutely no evidence to suggest that there is any correlation between walking age and intelligence.

2 Walking on tiptoes When children learn to walk they will normally walk on tiptoes for the first six months. However, a child who is still walking on tiptoes after six months should be seen by a doctor. There may be a problem involving the bones of the feet.

3 Walking with legs bowed or feet splayed outwards For the first year or two that they are walking young children often adopt rather unusual postures. Until they have learned how to hold themselves and balance themselves they will often walk with legs bent and sway from side to side rather alarmingly. This is nothing to worry about unless it persists after the age of 2.

4 Limping There are dozens of different reasons why children may limp. The problem causing the limp may be something as simple and trivial as a stone in the shoe, badly fitting shoes, or a painful verruca. It may be an injury to a joint or bone which has resulted from a fall or a blow. Or it may be a serious disorder such as an infection or dislocation affecting a major joint.

5 He walks with a strange gait If there is any muscular, skeletal or neurological malfunction then your child's ability to walk may be badly affected. If one leg is shorter than the other, for example, he'll obviously walk with a strange gait.

How do we make the diagnosis?

Look for the obvious problems first. The commonest cause of a walking difficulty in a child is a stone in his shoe. The next most common problems are painful verrucas and shoes that don't fit properly. If you have excluded these possibilities and your child's walking problem is not the consequence of some recent minor injury then you should seek medical attention in order to exclude more serious disorders. Skeletal problems, in particular, if found early can be treated very effectively. If left too long they may produce more lasting damage.

How do we prevent walking problems developing?

1 Small children do not need to wear shoes when indoors. Shoes only serve to protect the feet from hard or rough surfaces, from dirt and the cold. Small feet will develop more freely without shoes.
2 When you do buy shoes for your child make sure that you buy good-fitting shoes. See page 285.
3 Sleeping suits and stretch suits and bootees that are not big enough can damage the growing feet as effectively as ill-fitting shoes.
4 Teach your child to look after the skin of his feet. Make sure that the skin between the toes is properly dried after bathing. If any sore places develop examine the shoes to look for possible causes. If verrucas, corns or other disorders appear and cannot be dealt with effectively at home then seek professional help from a chiropodist or doctor.

Warts

What are they?

Warts are small growths on the skin that are caused by viruses. They can occur anywhere on the body. In children they occur most frequently on the soles of the feet when they are known as verrucas.

What causes them?

Warts are caused by viruses. All those old wives' tales about warts being transmitted by frogs and toads have yet to be substantiated. The virus involved stimulates the reproduction of skin cells. This can happen very quickly and warts sometimes appear almost overnight. The virus is the human papilloma virus.

Are they infectious?

The short answer to this question is 'yes'. But there is a lot of controversy about just how easily warts are transmitted. The general consensus of opinion seems to be that they still need to be regarded as infectious. Children with verrucas are usually told that they cannot go swimming. In fact, it seems safe enough for them to do so as long as they wear a waterproof dressing over the wart. The risks associated with an inability to swim properly far exceed the risks which can be directly associated with warts.

What can we do about them?

Leave them alone and most warts will disappear by themselves in six months or so. It is this fact which is responsible for the existence of so many marvellous tales about getting rid of warts by blowing on them nine times when the moon is full or touching each wart with a pea on the first day of a new moon. It's also said that you can try rubbing warts with a thread, a grain of wheat or stone and then leaving the thread, grain of wheat or stone at a crossroads. The first person to pick up the object will become the owner of the wart.

Among the most imaginative myths are those which suggest that you try setting fire to cobwebs on top of the wart, that you make a mole's nose bleed and let the blood drip on to the wart or that you stroke the warts with a tortoiseshell cat's tail in the month of May.

All this nonsense is good fun but there is no doubt that warts are a terrible nuisance and they can be most dispiriting. Young girls are always very upset about warts which are visible and both boys and girls may find verrucas (or plantar warts as they are also known) quite painful.

Most of the available remedies for warts contain salicylic acid. Whatever product you buy will need to be applied every day for several weeks. Do read the instructions carefully. And do make sure that you don't get any of the application on any part of the skin other than the wart. Don't try removing a wart surgically at home. They often bleed, they can get infected and you're likely to make a mess of it.

When do we need to see the doctor?

You should see the doctor without delay if a growth that you think is a wart changes colour, shape or size or bleeds. And if a persistently unsightly or painful wart doesn't respond to home treatment it may also be worthwhile seeking professional advice. Your family doctor may deal with the wart himself or he may arrange an appointment with a dermatologist.

What will the doctor do?

Doctors use various techniques to remove warts. Some remove them surgically while others remove them with the aid of liquid nitrogen or carbon dioxide snow. Warts are sometimes burned off by cautery.

Wax in the ears

What causes it?

The skin inside the ear contains a number of special glands which produce a waxy substance designed to trap dust and dirt. Unfortunately wax production in some people is a little too enthusiastic and the wax collects and may block the canal which leads down to the ear drum. This accumulation of wax is probably the commonest cause of temporary deafness in adults although it is rather less common in children.

How do we make the diagnosis?

Wax that has built up into a blockage may produce pain and cause deafness. If you can see wax around the entrance to the ear then you won't have much difficulty in making this particular diagnosis.

What can we do about it?

You can remove wax that is visible with a cotton bud. Do not try removing wax that is out of sight. You are quite likely to push the wax deeper into the ear and to make it more difficult to get out. You are also likely to damage the drum if you use a sharp object such as a knitting needle. One expert I know always says that parents should never put anything smaller than their feet into their children's ears and I think he's right.

When should we see the doctor?
You should see the doctor if you suspect that your child has wax accumulating deep inside the ear canal.

What will the doctor do?
He will either remove the wax with a special probe or else he will prescribe drops which will soften the wax. These drops sometimes bring the wax out by themselves. The drops will certainly make it easier to remove the wax by syringing. The doctor simply squirts warm water into the ear canal and washes out the wax. There is no real need to remove wax unless it is causing pain or deafness.

Weight loss

What causes it?
When a child loses weight there are a number of possible causes. Before looking for a cause, however, it is important to check that there has actually been a real weight loss and not just a change in the child's shape. Up to the age of about nine months babies have a good deal of subcutaneous fat and tend to look fairly plump. After that age most babies lose some of their fat and begin to look thinner and more muscular. The baby who looked rather chubby may begin to look rather lean. Ribs which were once hidden may become apparent for the first time. Be certain that your child is actually losing weight and not just growing up and changing shape.

If a genuine weight loss has been discovered there are a number of possible causes. These causes can be grouped into one of three major categories.

1 There isn't enough food going into the child
    (a) A breast feeding mother may not be making enough milk.
    (b) The teat on a bottle may not be large enough.
    (c) The bottle may be presented in such a way that the baby cannot drink from it properly. If, for example, the teat is

placed underneath the tongue then the baby is going to have a lot of difficulty in gaining any nourishment from the bottle.

(d) Children who vomit a good deal may lose weight. Sometimes vomiting merely results from the fact that too much wind is being swallowed with food. Occasionally vomiting is caused by a blockage which prevents food going down into the stomach.

(e) Children in their second year often discover that they can control their parents by refusing to eat. The more the parents try to force the child to eat the more the child will refuse and demand more love and attention.

(f) If a child is offered a huge plateful of unappetising-looking food he may turn away in despair.

(g) A child who has a sore or infected mouth may not eat well. Sore teeth, infected gums and thrush are three common problems.

2 The food that is going into your child isn't being absorbed properly

(a) If a child has persistent diarrhoea then however much food is being eaten the chances are that weight will be lost. Diarrhoea may be associated with an intestinal infection or a malabsorption syndrome in which the child's intestinal mucosa is unable to extract the proper nourishment from the food that is passing through.

(b) Even where there isn't any diarrhoea a child who is losing weight may have a malabsorption problem.

(c) If there is a congenital abnormality in the gastrointestinal tract then food will not be properly absorbed (see Hirschprung's Disease, page 261).

3 An internal problem which means that the food that's going in isn't enough

(a) A child who is suffering from undiagnosed diabetes mellitus will often lose weight as the disease progresses. Diabetes mellitus is discussed on page 108.

(b) In the adrenogenital syndrome hormone deficiencies result in changes within the body which may include a failure to gain weight.

(c) Severe infections may result in food being burned up at

such a rate that even the child who seems to be eating well will lose weight.

How do we make the diagnosis?

If your child is losing weight (and isn't on a weight-reducing diet of course!) and the diagnosis is not obvious then you should not try to make a diagnosis yourself. There are so many potentially serious disorders which can produce a weight loss but which can be treated effectively when tackled early that you shouldn't delay in seeking advice. Weight loss is a symptom that needs to be taken seriously.

What will the doctor do?

He'll arrange for whatever investigations are necessary to find out why your child is losing weight. Then he'll treat the underlying problem.

Wheezing

What is it?

When we breathe in and out the air moves along the passageways within the lungs quite silently. There is no reason for any noise because the tubes through which the air passes are wide enough to allow the air to move quite freely and slowly. If those passages become narrowed for any reason then the air will have difficulty in getting in and out of the lungs. It will make a noise as it does so. That's a wheeze.Try whistling with your mouth wide open and then with your lips pursed tightly together and you'll see what I mean.

What causes it?

Anything that makes the internal air passages narrower will cause a wheeze. A chest infection may cause wheezing, as can the inhalation of any small foreign body which is blocking part of the respiratory system.

By far the commonest cause of wheezing, however, is asthma. Asthma is discussed at greater length on page 33.

What can we do about it?

If a child's wheezing is made worse by an allergy then it will help if you can isolate the child from the allergen or if you can arrange for desensitising injections. When the allergy cannot be identified then it will usually help if nylon or cotton bed linen and clothes are preferred to wool. Feather pillows should be avoided and all dust should be cleaned away regularly and quite obsessionally. It is wiser not to have pets or to at least keep them out of the house.

The quality of the air can also affect wheezing. Cold air, very dry air, air polluted by cigarette smoke and by cooking or heating with gas can all make wheezing worse.

Worry and emotional upsets are also an important factor in the production of wheezing. If a child's wheezing gets worse for no reason at all it may be worthwhile trying to make sure that there are no problems at school that you do not know about.

There are no drugs or medicines that can be bought over the counter that I recommend for the wheezing child. But there are some very effective drugs available on prescription. If your child is given one of these do make sure that you know whether the drug has been prescribed to prevent wheezing or to cure it. And do make sure that you keep a supply of medicine in stock. Wheezing attacks invariably seem to start during the night or on bank holidays and you'll save a lot of time if you have a small emergency stock of medicine locked away.

Finally, don't be tempted to wrap a wheezy child in cotton wool. Over protected children tend to suffer more because they start worrying themselves. There is no reason why a wheezy child shouldn't lead a perfectly normal, active life whenever his wheezing is under control.

When do we need to see the doctor?

Unless it is a purely temporary problem and seems of little practical significance wheezing should always be assessed by a doctor. If a wheezy child is breathless then contact should be made with some urgency.

Whooping cough

What causes it?

An organism called bordetella pertussis is usually responsible for the development of whooping cough. The infection is transmitted in droplets and caught when a child breathes in germs coughed out by another victim.

How common is it?
Whooping cough tends to come in epidemics. It is a moderately common infection of childhood.

Is it infectious?
Yes. The incubation period is usually between one and two weeks.

How do we make the diagnosis?
To begin with the symptoms usually suggest that a cold is starting. Your child will have a runny nose and a cough. There is not usually much of a fever. However, the cough will gradually get worse and worse and after two or three weeks your child will probably begin to 'whoop' every time he coughs. The character-istic 'whooping' noise occurs when the patient breathes in. At this stage vomiting is usually also a problem.

The coughing is usually worse at night and is often brought on when the sufferer sits down to eat.

When do we need to see the doctor?
If your child is run down or under 3 years of age then you should call or see your doctor as soon as you suspect whooping cough. However, if your child is normally healthy and fit and is more than 3 years old then there is not any real need to call for medical advice unless the symptoms are particularly troublesome or are worrying. Antibiotics are only usually necessary if there is an added chest infection.

What can we do about it?
Children with whooping cough should be kept away from school for between four and six weeks and they should also be kept away from babies and older people. The disease can cause serious problems at both ends of the age spectrum – but particularly among babies.

If your child coughs a lot he may find it easier to breathe if he remains half sitting rather than lying down. If he vomits every time he tries to eat give him small portions of food that he can easily chew and swallow. Unless your child is obviously too ill it is also well worth remembering that fresh air is good for a whooping cough victim.

What about the whooping cough vaccination?

The whooping cough vaccine provides some protection against the disease. There can be problems with the vaccine so read the notes on page 308 and discuss your own child's suitability for vaccination with your general practitioner.

Wind

What is it?

Air sometimes gets into the stomach and from the stomach manages to find its way along the rest of the intestine. Bubbles of air which have collected in the intestinal tract are usually known collectively as wind.

What causes it?

We all tend to swallow a little air whenever we feed and babies who haven't graduated to solids are more likely than children or adults to do this because they take most of their food in by sucking.

When a bottle fed baby develops a good deal of wind then there are several possible causes. If the bottle is nearly empty and the baby is still sucking then the milk is obviously going to be mixed with air. If the opening in the teat is too small or too large there is a similar risk.

It is also possible for a baby to swallow a good deal of air if he cries. Crying is said to cause wind more often than wind causes crying.

What can we do about it?

There isn't any need to do very much at all about the baby who has accumulated a little too much air. If the air passes all the way along the intestinal tract some of it will be absorbed and some of it will pass out at the other end.

I appreciate, however, that the majority of mothers will feel better if they manage to empty the wind out of their babies after feeding. 'Burping' is an accepted way of life in many parts of the world.

To encourage air to come up out of the stomach you don't have
to manoeuvre your baby into any unusual positions. All you really
have to do is to remember that air will come up more easily if the
baby is held upright. Lying your baby down straight after a feed
is likely to cause problems if there is any air trapped in the
stomach because the bubble of gas just won't be able to move.

Many babies bring up a little milk together with the wind. This
isn't anything to worry about.

When do we need to see the doctor?
If the problem is simply wind then you don't need medical advice
unless you can't work out why your baby is swallowing too much
air. If you aren't certain that the problem is wind, or if your baby
seems to be in any pain, then you should ask for medical advice.

Worms

What are they?
Most of us are familiar only with the sort of worms which wriggle
about in the garden and serve as luncheon for the birds. There
are, however, a number of variations on this common or garden
theme and some of these variations live as parasites inside human
beings.

I have listed below some of the worms most likely to find a
home in your child's intestinal tract.

1 Threadworms (enterobius vermicularis) Also known as pin-
worms, these are the commonest of all the parasitic worms. They
are found all over the world, are said to affect one in three of all
children and are most frequently found in children between the
ages of 5 and 9. Looking like tiny cotton threads, they are about 1
cm long.

The worms pair in the intestines and the eggs are passed in the
patient's stools. Because the anus itches the patient scratches that
region and picks up some eggs on his fingers. The eggs then get
back into the intestines either through contaminated food or
through the fingers being sucked.

2 Roundworms (ascaris lumbricoides) These look like and are
about the same size as the ordinary common earthworm. To

begin with a child swallows a fertilised egg which hatches out in the upper part of the intestine. The larva burrows through the intestinal wall, enters a vein and is carried first into the heart and then into the lungs.

In the lungs the larva causes an infection which makes the child cough. The larva is then duly coughed up in the sputum and swallowed so that it gets back into the intestine. There it develops into an adult worm.

3 Hook worms (ankylostoma duodenale and necator americanus) This type of worm is very common in tropical countries. The worms are about 1 cm long and they live in the duodenum. Their eggs pass along the intestinal tract and hatch out into larvae in the outside world. These larvae then find their way into the skin of the next human being with whom they can make contact. They make their way to the heart, then to the lungs and then into the intestinal tract where they make their home in the duodenum.

4 Trichinosis (trichinella spiralis) This very small, round worm normally lives in a pig's intestines but the embryo worms move out of the intestines and into the muscles to develop. If the inadequately cooked meat of an infected pig is eaten the worm develops in a human host instead of a pig.

5 Tapeworms (taenia saginata, taenia solium, diphyllobothrium latum) The adult tapeworm can be several metres long and about 1 cm wide. Tapeworms have a very complicated life cycle which is a tribute to the ingenuity of nature. Adult tapeworms live in the intestines of human beings but their eggs pass out in the faeces of that host. If those eggs are then swallowed by what is known as an intermediate host (taenia saginata uses cattle as an inter-mediate host, taenia solium uses pigs and diphyllobothrium latum uses fish) the larvae will hatch out and get into the muscles of that host. Then, if the infected meat is eaten the cycle can begin again.

Tapeworms have tiny heads with which they attach themselves to the duodenum. They are said to look like long pieces of ribbon.

6 Whipworm (trichuris trichura) A worm of some 3-5 cm in length which is found all over the world. Its eggs are found in the host's faeces and from there find their way into a fresh host.

7 Toxocara (toxocara canis, toxocara catis) These two parasitic worms normally live in dogs and cats. They spread to human beings more by accident than by design. Normally the eggs are passed in the faeces and then picked up by another dog or cat but young children who play in grass that has been soiled by dogs and cats or who touch and fondle domestic animals are quite likely to acquire the worms themselves.

The larvae of these worms can move into the liver, the central nervous system and the eyes and they can cause serious damage.

Are they infectious?
The short answer is 'yes' – all these worms are infectious in that they can be passed on from one individual sufferer to another. Children are more susceptible to some worms because their standard of personal hygiene tends to be lower.

Threadworms, roundworms and toxocara are the three types of worm most commonly passed on in this way. Threadworms are the commonest of all and toxocara are the most serious.

How do we make the diagnosis?
Threadworms are probably the type of worms your child is most likely to contract. Frequently there won't be any symptoms at all and unless you happen to notice the typical small, white threadlike worms in the stools you won't know that your child even has them. When symptoms do occur the most common problem is itching around the anus. This is invariably worse at night. The itching is sometimes so severe that it results in disturbed sleep. Some general practitioners claim that if a child complains of an itchy bottom at night then the diagnosis is worms until proved otherwise.

A child who has roundworms may present with all sorts of different symptoms ranging from vomiting and coughing to strange, inexplicable abdominal pains. A child who has hookworm will usually have an itchy and inflamed spot on the skin where the larva entered and diarrhoea and weight loss are the two most usual general symptoms. Tapeworms, despite their size and length, sometimes produce no symptoms at all. When there are symptoms diarrhoea, abdominal pains and an unusual hunger are the three most commonly mentioned.

The other worms I've mentioned are relatively difficult to diagnose without doing special tests. The symptoms tend to be vague and persistent and non-specifc.

How do we stop our children getting worms?

1 Ensure that your children wash their hands after every visit to the lavatory.

2 If you have a dog or a cat make sure that the animal is regularly examined and treated if it has worms. Puppies are more likely to have worms than adult dogs.

What can we do about it?

If you decide that your child has threadworms or roundworms then you may be able to treat the problem yourself. The most useful drug is piperazine. You should be able to buy this without a doctor's prescription. Do follow the manufacturer's instructions carefully.

It used to be said that if a child had threadworms or roundworms then the rest of the household should be treated as though they also had worms. I don't agree with this.

Should you suspect that your child has any other form of worm then you should ask your doctor for advice.

What is it?
A glossary of common children's diseases

These are intended as introductory notes only. I have not included any details of incidence, treatment or prognosis in this section.

Albinism There is an absence of pigment in the skin, hair and eyes. This failure of melanin production means that the skin will burn very easily in the sun.

Anoxia A low level of oxygen in the blood and tissues.

Anuria A failure to produce any urine at all.

Arachnodactyly The fingers and toes are abnormally long. There may also be problems affecting the eyes and the heart.

Ascites An abnormal collection of fluid within the abdominal cavity.

Asphyxia A condition in which the tissues do not receive enough oxygen – as in suffocation.

Ataxia A defect in part of the brain usually producing a tremor and unsteady gait.

Atelectasis A failure of the lungs to expand.

Athetosis The child with athetosis will move involuntarily either in a slow, writhing way or in jerky movements. These involuntary movements disappear when the child is asleep.

Atresia The absence of a normal opening or passageway.

Atrial septal defect A type of congenital heart disease.

Atrophy When a part of the body which has developed quite normally shrinks it is said to atrophy.

Autism A little understood psychiatric disorder affecting children. Some doctors describe autism as a type of schizophrenic disease. Others deny that it exists as a clinical entity. Affected children fail to react normally and seem unable to develop normal relationships.

Bronchiectasis The passages of the lung are infected and greatly enlarged.

Bronchiolitis Inflammation of the smaller passageways in the lungs.

Bronchitis Inflammation of the larger passageways in the lungs.

Bronchopneumonia Inflammation of the larger passageways in the lungs and the lung tissue itself.

Cancer Also known as carcinoma. A general term used to describe any malignant tumour. Cancer cells multiply rapidly and are often badly formed. Some cancers are deadly but many are curable.

Cataract An opacity of the lens of the eye. In children cataracts are usually caused by an infection or a nutritional deficiency.

Cerebral palsy A permanent disorder of posture and movement caused by a brain defect.

Chorea Also known as Sydenham's chorea and St Vitus's dance. Children with chorea fidget, drop things and sigh a good deal. They have many involuntary movements which may include facial grimaces. Many children with chorea previously suffered from rheumatic fever.

Chromosomal abnormalities Some of the most obvious chromosomal abnormalities affect the sex chromosomes. A normal female has two X chromosomes while a normal male has an X and a Y chromosome. Occasionally children are born with three X chromosomes, two X and Y chromosomes or a single sex chromosome.

Cirrhosis Usually refers to an inflammatory disorder affecting the liver.

Club foot Also known as talipes. If the foetus is stuck in an abnormal position while in the uterus the foot may be deformed. This is the commonest cause of a club foot although there are children with talipes caused by developmental malformations.

Coeliac disease An enzyme defect in the intestinal wall means that the child with coeliac disease cannot tolerate the protein gluten which is present in wheat and rye flour. Gluten-free foods must be eaten for life. Until diagnosed a child with this disease will usually be underweight, miserable and suffer from a distended abdomen, vomiting and diarrhoea.

Cold sores Blisters caused by herpes which usually occur on or around the lips.

Colitis An inflammation of the colon.

Congenital disorder Any abnormality present at birth. A congenital disorder may be a result of an inherited problem or a factor operative during pregnancy.

Coryza A common cold.

Cot deaths This problem is as yet unexplained. Every year a number of infants are found dead in their cots. No apparent cause is found.

Cretinism If there is no thyroid gland or the thyroid gland is not producing enough thyroid hormone the child's metabolic processes will be extremely slow. Growth will be retarded, the facial features will be coarse, the skin cold, the tongue large, the abdomen pot-bellied, the hair dry and brittle. Treatment with thyroid hormones will produce a miraculous recovery.

Croup A difficulty in breathing usually associated with laryngeal spasm.

Cryptorchidism An undescended testis or testes.

Cyanosis A bluish tinge to the skin caused by a lack of oxygen.

Cystic fibrosis Also known as fibrocystic disease of the pancreas although that name is rather misleading since mucus-producing glands elsewhere around the body may be involved. An inherited enzyme defect seems to be responsible and the distended mucous glands produce dilatation which is followed by obstruction and fibrosis. The lungs, liver and intestines may be affected.

Deaf mute A child who can neither talk nor hear.

Diphtheria An infection which usually affects the throat or the throat and nose. A grey membrane is produced by the bacilli involved and usually spreads over the tonsils.

Down's syndrome Also known as mongolism. There are four types of Down's syndrome but all are caused by a chromosomal abnormality. In the commonest variation the patient has forty-seven chromosomes instead of forty-six. Mongols get their name from the fact that their slanting eyes suggest an oriental appearance but all patients so called are mentally defective.

Dwarfism Any condition in which a child fails to grow to average size. The opposite to dwarfism is gigantism. Dwarfism may be caused by disorders affecting the development of bones, by hormonal disorders, by infections, by metabolic disorders or by nutritional problems.

Dysentery An inflammation of the large intestine characterised by diarrhoea and by the passage of blood.

Dyspnoea Difficult breathing.

Emphysema The abnormal presence of air in body tissues.

Empyema The presence of pus within the cavity around the lungs.

Encephalitis An inflammation of the brain.

Encopresis Faecal incontinence.

Enuresis Incontinence of urine during sleep.

Epispadias Congenital malformation in which the upper wall of the urethra is absent. In males it means that the urethral opening is located on the side of the penis instead of at the end.

Erythema Redness of the skin.

Extradural haematoma If blood vessels within the skull are injured bleeding outside the brain may occur and put pressure on the brain. An extradural haematoma can be caused by even apparently slight head injuries. Signs to look for are headache, vomiting, restlessness or drowsiness.

Friedreich's ataxia A hereditary, degenerative disorder affecting the brain and spinal cord. Children with this disorder tend to have indistinct speech and to be unsteady on their feet.

Gastroenteritis An inflammation of the stomach and the intestines.

Genetic disorders Genes are the individual units of material within chromosomes which carry hereditary characteristics. A genetic problem is, therefore, one which has been inherited.

Gigantism Part of the pituitary gland overproduces growth hormone. Growth starts usually early in childhood and continues for longer than usual.

Glaucoma Excessive pressure inside the eye which can cause pain and blindness.

Glomerulonephritis An infection affecting the tissues of the kidneys.

Goitre Enlargement of the thyroid gland.

Guillain Barré syndrome Also known as acute infective polyneuritis. A viral disorder producing muscle weakness and tenderness.

Gynaecomastia Overdevelopment of the breasts in the male.

Haemangioma A benign lesion made up of blood vessels.

Haematoma A clot of blood in body tissues.

Haematuria Blood in the urine.

Haemolytic disease of the newborn An unusually rapid breakdown of blood cells in a baby which may be produced if maternal and foetal blood groups are incompatible.

Haemophilia An inherited disorder in which a factor essential for blood clotting is absent. Minor injuries can cause severe bleeding. Bleeding that occurs into joints can produce crippling.

Hemiparesis A slight or incomplete paralysis affecting one side of the body.

Hemiplegia A paralysis of one side of the body.

Henoch-Schönlein purpura Also known as anaphylactoid purpura. Usually follows a throat or chest infection. A typical rash on the buttocks and limbs is usually accompanied by limb pains and may be accompanied by kidney infection.

Hepatitis An inflammation of the liver.

Hermaphroditism A condition in which an individual has both ovarian and testicular tissue.

Herpes A skin disease characterised by the development of small vesicles. There may be a considerable amount of pain.

Hirschprung's disease Constipation and abdominal distension are common symptoms in this condition in which nerves to the large bowel are missing.

Hodgkin's disease Also known as lymphadenoma. Lymph nodes swell and become firm when this tumour develops.

Hydrocephalus An excessive amount of cerebrospinal fluid produces a raised pressure within the skull. If the condition starts early in life the head may be greatly enlarged.

Hydrocoele A collection of fluid around the testis and within the scrotum.

Hypertension An abnormally increased blood pressure.

Hyperthyroidism An overactive thyroid gland producing too much thyroid hormone.

Hypoglycaemia A low blood sugar.

Hypospadias A developmental error which means that in boys the urethra opens on the side of the penis instead of the end.

Hypotension A low blood pressure.

Hypothermia A low body temperature.

Hypotonia A diminished strength or tension in the muscles.

Hypoxia A low level of oxygen in the body.

Hysteria A condition in which an anxious patient will exaggerate problems and may appear to have a lack of control over emotional feelings. The hysteric may behave irrationally and may appear to have any one of a number of genuine disorders.

Icterus Jaundice.

Idiocy Severe mental deficiency which renders a child incapable of looking after himself. The IQ of an idiot will be less than 25.

Ileus Intestinal obstruction.

Infantilism A failure to develop properly.

Intertrigo Chafing and redness of the skin which usually occurs where two folds of skin rub together.

Intussusception One piece of bowel slides inside another piece of bowel – in the same way that you can push a glove finger inside itself.

Iritis An inflammation of the iris in the eye.

Ischaemia An interruption of the blood supply means that an area of body tissue is temporarily deprived of blood.

Keratosis The formation of bony growth.

Kernicterus A severe form of jaundice which affects babies and which involves the brain and spinal cord.

Kwashiorkor A disease which is widespread in developing countries and which is caused by lack of protein. Growth slows down, the skin becomes dry and the legs swell.

Kyphosis A round deformity of the back.

Labial adhesions The labia minora are stuck together. They can usually be parted without difficulty.

Lanuge The fine hair that can be found on a newborn baby.

Lead poisoning Lethargy, abdominal pain, vomiting and loss of appetite are the commonest symptoms. Children used to acquire lead poisoning from sucking toys decorated with lead paint. Today, however, children are more at risk from atmospheric lead pollution caused by motor cars using petrol rich in lead.

Leukaemia A disorder in which the number of leucocytes in the blood increases rapidly and uncontrollably.

Lipoma A fatty lump or tumour.

Marasmus Progressive wasting or failure to thrive.

Mastisis Inflammation of the breast tissue.

Mastoiditis Inflammation of the space in the portion of temporal bone lying behind the meatus of the ear.

Masturbation Self-stimulation of the genital organs. A normal activity among children of all ages.

Meckel's diverticulum An extra piece of bowel with a blind ending. Pain and bleeding can develop.

Meconium Dark green material which comes from the intestines of a newborn baby.

Melaena Blood in the faeces produces darkening. Sometimes the faeces will be quite black and sticky.

Meningioma A tumour of the brain.

Meningitis Inflammation of the meninges (the membranes which surround the brain and spinal cord).

Meningocoele A protrusion of the meninges through a defect in the vertebral column or the skull.

Mesenteric adenitis Inflammation of the glands in the membrane which attaches the intestine to the posterior abdominal wall.

Microcephaly An abnormally small head.

Mongolism See Down's syndrome.

Moniliasis See thrush.

Muscular dystrophy Various disorders come within this general category. In all the main difficulty is muscular weakness. The basic problem lies in the development of the muscles themselves.

Myasthenia gravis The passage of messages between nerves and muscles is disturbed. The eye muscles are usually the first ones affected. Then the muscles of the mouth and throat are affected with the result that speech and swallowing are disturbed.

Myelocoele Spina bifida with protrusion of the spinal cord through the opening.

Myeloma A tumour made up of cells which normally exist only in bone marrow.

Myocarditis Inflammation of the heart muscle.

Myopia Short-sightedness.

Naevus A small flat tumour of the skin which may or may not be pigmented and may or may not be hairy.

Nephritis Inflammation of the kidney.

Nephrosis Any disease affecting the kidney.

Nephrotic syndrome Oedema is the most common symptom of this condition in which the kidney is the organ basically involved. Protein and blood may appear in the urine and the blood pressure may rise. There are a number of causes for the nephrotic syndrome.

Neuritis An inflammation of a nerve.

Neurofibromatosis Also known as von Recklinghausen's disease. Brown spots and small lumps may appear on the skin. There may be bony problems and mental retardation too.

Nystagmus A continuous rolling movement of the eyeball.

Oedema An abnormal collection of fluid in the body.

Oliguria A reduction in the amount of urine being passed.

Oophoritis Inflammation of an ovary.

Ophthalmia neonatorum Also known as conjunctivitis or sticky eye. One or both eyes are infected and the lids are stuck together with pus.

Orchitis Inflammation of a testis.

Osteoarthritis A degenerative joint disease.

Osteomyelitis Inflammation of bone caused by a small organism.

Pancreatitis Inflammation of the pancreas.

Papilloedema Swelling of the optic disc.

Paraphimosis The foreskin is pulled back behind the glans penis and cannot be moved.

Paraplegia Paralysis of half of the body – usually the lower half.

Paronychia Infection of the tissues next to a nail.

Parotitis Inflammation of the parotid gland.

Paul Bunnell test Test for glandular fever.

Peri-anal excoriation Soreness around the anus can develop after diarrhoea – particularly when a baby is being fed on cows' milk. A barrier cream will prevent the condition developing.

Periodic syndrome There are various forms for this syndrome. The commonest is probably cyclical vomiting in which vomiting attacks recur. Sometimes the main symptom is recurrent abdominal pain. The only thing that the various manifestations have in common is that they come and go according to a predictable pattern and that between attacks the child is quite well.

Peritonitis Inflammation of the membrane lining the abdominal walls.

Pertussis Whooping cough.

Pes planus Flat foot.

Petchiae A small red spot caused by the effusion of blood.

Pharyngitis Inflammation of the pharynx.

Phimosis The foreskin is tight and cannot be drawn back.

Phocomelia A baby with phocomelia is born with hands and feet but no arms or legs. Thalidomide produced babies with phocomelia.

Photophobia An inability to tolerate light.

Pica A craving for unnatural food substances.

Pigeon chest Forward protrusion of the sternum can be caused by bone problems, asthma or heart disease.

Pleural effusion Fluid in the pleural cavity. (The pleura is the membrane which covers the lungs and lines the chest.)

Pleurisy Inflammation of the pleura.

Pneumonia Inflammation of the lung caused by an infection.

Pneumothorax The presence of air or gas in the pleural cavity.

Poliomyelitis An infectious disease caused by a virus. Sufferers may become partly or completely paralysed. A vaccine provides effective protection.

Polyarthritis Inflammation of several joints.

Polydactyly The presence of too many fingers or toes.

Polydipsia Excessive thirst and drinking of water.

Polyneuritis Inflammation of a number of nerves.

Polyp A smooth round nodule on a stalk which projects into the central space of a hollow organ.

Polyuria The passage of excessive amounts of urine.

Premature infant Officially any baby whose birth weight is less than $5\frac{1}{2}$ lb ($2\frac{1}{2}$ kg) is premature. (This means that a baby born at full term may still be 'premature' while a baby born early may not officially fit the definition required for a 'premature baby'.) Premature babies often need special care since they tend to be particularly susceptible to infection.

Prickly heat Heat rash.

Psoriasis The skin produces new cells too quickly. A superficial layer of flaky white cells covers a red, raw area. Psoriasis can be inherited and may be triggered by stress.

Purpura Small purple patches on the skin and mucous membranes.

Pyaemia The presence of pus in the blood.

Pyelitis Inflammation of the kidney pelvis (the area where the ureter joins the kidneys).

Pyelonephritis Inflammation of the kidneys and kidney pelvis.

Pyloric stenosis Vomiting develops in the second or third week of life. The patient remains very hungry but brings back everything he eats. There is hypertrophy of the muscles at the bottom of the oesophagus and food cannot get through.

Pyrexia Fever.

Quadriplegia Also known as tetraplegia. Paralysis of all four limbs.

Quinsy Inflammation, infection and swelling of the tonsil and surrounding tissue.

Rheumatic fever The joints and heart are affected by changes caused by a streptococcal infection. Rheumatic fever usually follows a throat infection.

Rickets An abnormality of bone development caused by a lack of vitamin D.

Scarlet fever Streptococcus causes this disease which consists of a rash and pharyngitis. There is usually a fever, loss of appetite and vomiting.

Scleroderma The skin becomes thickened due to the deposition of extra collagen fibres. Contractures develop and the face becomes immobile.

Scoliosis A lateral curvature of the spine.

Scurvy Disorder resulting from a lack of vitamin C. Bleeding commonly occurs into the skin and into joints. The gums become spongy and swollen.

Sickle cell disease Red cells only survive for fifteen to sixty days instead of the normal 120 days. There is anaemia and the spleen enlarges as the marrow attempts to produce enough new cells to compensate. Children with sickle cell anaemia are usually underdeveloped with thin limbs.

Spasticity The muscles are held in permanent spasm.

Spider naevi These look like small red spiders and are usually of no significance.

Spina bifida A bony defect in the arch of one or more spinal vertebrae may be of no significance but may be associated with an abnormality of the meninges or spinal cord. In severe cases the spinal canal is laid open.

Splenomegaly Enlarged spleen.

Still's disease Acute rheumatoid arthritis in children.

Stomatitis Inflammation of the mucosa in the mouth.

Strabismus Squint.

Stridor A harsh and shrill sound.

Sydenham's chorea See page 257.

Syndactyly The fingers or toes are joined together.

Syphilis, congenital If a mother has syphilis then her baby can be born with syphilis.

Tachycardia Abnormally fast heart rate.

Talipes Club foot. See page 257.

Telengiectasia Small red lesions in the skin or mucous membranes caused by dilated capillaries.

Tenesmus Painful, unproductive straining to open the bowels or empty the bladder.

Teratoma A tumour consisting of different types of cell.

Tetanus Spasms caused by an organism entering the body through a dirty cut or lesion of some kind. Can be prevented by vaccination.

Tetany Muscle twitchings, cramps and convulsions caused by abnormal calcium metabolism.

Thrombocytopenia A fall in the number of platelets in the blood.

Thrombosis Blood clot.

Thrush Fungal infection which usually affects the mouth or the vagina. The infection appears as white patches on the mucous membranes.

Thyrotoxicosis Condition caused by an overactive thyroid gland.

Toxoplasmosis A protozoan infection which can affect the brain, eye and liver. Can be contracted by eating infected food or coming into contact with infected animals or their faeces. Can be acquired congenitally.

Tuberculosis An infection which can present in many different ways. All children should be tested for tuberculosis while at school.

Uraemia An accumulation in the blood of toxic substances normally excreted in the urine. Symptoms include nausea, vomiting and convulsions. May be caused by nephritis.

Urticaria Red, itchy rash. Also known as nettle rash.

Varicella Chickenpox.

Variola Smallpox.

Vesicle
1 A fluid containing blister.
2 A bladder like cavity.

Vitiligo Patches of depigmented skin occur for no known reason.

Vulvitis Inflammation of the vulva.

Home care

I'm a great believer in home medical care.

If you know how to look after your children you and they will benefit in a number of very specific ways.

1 Not only are the majority of simple, uncomplicated disorders best treated at home but symptomatic home remedies are often cheaper, safer and just as effective as more powerful and potentially hazardous modern solutions.

2 Learn to look after your children whenever you can and you will be able to offer a far better service than any professional could hope to provide for the simple but vital reason that you will be *there* all the time. Learn to look for the imporant warning signs and learn to be aware of when you need professional assistance and you'll be able to offer help, support and comfort quite safely.

3 The more you understand what causes symptoms and how they can be relieved the more you will understand just how to take advantage of professional medical care.

4 Finally, there is the undeniable fact that although doctors try not to become blasé when patients cry wolf and repeatedly ask for help with minor problems there is risk that those parents who are always calling for assistance will get less-than-perfect service when they really need medical help.

The home medicine chest

Every home should have a medicine cabinet which is properly stocked. Ideally, your medicine cabinet should have a lock on it so that the medicines inside it can be kept out of the reach of small children. Although medicine cabinets are traditionally kept in the bathroom this isn't really the best place for drugs. The variations in temperature which can occur there may accelerate the rate at which drugs deteriorate. Any room which has a more or less stable temperature is more suitable.

Before stocking up with suitable home remedies clear out all the half-empty, improperly labelled bottles which have accumulated over the years. Anything that is not clearly labelled should be thrown away. Discard all medicines that are more than six months old. (Calamine lotion and menthol crystals can be kept longer.) Tablets and medicines can be flushed down the lavatory.

It doesn't cost much to stock a basic home medicine cabinet. You can keep the cost right down by buying non-branded products.

Your medicine cabinet should contain:

1 A pain reliever such as soluble aspirin or paracetamol. The doses for children should be on the bottles.

2 A hot-water bottle. Wrapped in a pillow case or thin towel a hot water bottle can be held against a painful ear, bruised joint or aching abdomen. It will often provide considerable comfort and relief.

3 A kaolin mixture for the relief of simple diarrhoea.

4 A bottle of calamine lotion to help with itchy spots and rashes.

5 An inhalant. A small bottle of menthol crystals will last for a long time and can be used to relieve catarrh and sinus troubles.

6 A laxative. Bran is the simplest and safest – and the only one suitable for children.

7 A small bottle of liquid antiseptic.

8 Zinc and castor oil ointment – for nappy rashes.

9 A teething ring (if appropriate).

10 A small bottle of olive oil – for removing foreign bodies from the ears.

11 For motion sickness, a small bottle of promethazine tablets.

12 If you want to include a gripe mixture I suggest you use a product containing dicyclomine hydrochloride.

13 An ordinary glass and mercury thermometer.

14 Whatever bandages you can use without tying yourself up in knots.

15 A measuring spoon or glass for liquid medicines.

16 A small packet of cotton wool.

17 A tin of assorted fabric plasters.

18 Any necessary prescription drugs.

Basic home nursing tips

1 Few patients need to stay in bed all day. Unless your child's doctor has given instructions to the contrary your child should certainly be able to get out of bed to bathe and use the toilet. Most children feel much better if they're allowed to get up, watch television or sit in a chair and play.

2 If you do have to look after a patient who is going to be bed-bound for a long time try and get hold of a hospital-type bed. If you have to bend over an ordinary divan bed you'll soon get a bad back!

3 Sick rooms quickly get very stuffy so don't be afraid to have a window open. Stale air is good for germs, not convalescent patients.

4 Crisp, clean bed sheets are extremely soothing. Try and change sheets as often as you can.

5 Powdering with talc helps prevent the development of sore places.

6 Unless your doctor has specifically forbidden exercise encourage your child to exercise regularly. A rubber ball is good for strengthening the fingers and hand muscles. Toe wriggling keeps the feet fit.

7 If your child needs to take drugs of any kind keep a chart by the bedside and tick off pills and medicines as they're taken. That way you won't be left wondering whether or not you've given the right dose at the right time. Read the notes on prescribed drugs on page 301.

8 Fill a vacuum flask with an iced drink and keep it by the bedside.

9 Children who are ill often have poor appetites. Try and make food as attractive as possible. Don't put too much on the plate at once and remember that weak patients often cope better with foods that don't need too much cutting or chewing.

10 If you need to take your child's temperature first put the thermometer into cold water and dry it carefully. Then put it either in the mouth or an armpit (held in position by putting the arm on that side across the chest). Don't take his temprature after your child has just had a wash or a hot drink. Leave the thermometer in position for a minimum of three minutes.

11 Give your young patient things to look forward to. Point out good programmes on the TV or radio. Tell him in advance if you've got something special for him to eat.

12 Keep a few puzzles, toys, magazines or books on one side for the dull moments.

13 If your child is in a room away from the parts of the house where you'll be working try and fix up some sort of communications system with telephones. Otherwise prepare a two-way system with tin cans and bits of string. Failing all else a walking stick that can be banged on the floor will have to do!

14 Keep an eye on the visitors who call. Young patients can easily get tired. Don't let too many people into the sick room.

15 Don't get too professional! Make sure that you find time occasionally to just sit down and chat or play a game.

Quick reference home nursing: *specific tips*

Aching joints Wrap a warm towel around the affected joint – or try putting a hot-water bottle (wrapped in a thin towel) next to the joint.

Bad breath As a short-term solution try chewing a sprig of parsley – or a fairly vigorous tooth cleaning session.

Boils Put a warm compress on top of the boil – or hold a well-wrapped hot-water bottle nearby.

Burns and scalds Keep the burnt area in cold water for as long as possible – five minutes at least.

Catarrh A child with a stuffy nose or with catarrh will be helped by a long steamy bath. If your child can't sleep because of catarrh fill a flask with hot water and a menthol crystal – he can take a sniff in the night if he awakes all 'blocked up'.

Cold hands Get him to whirl his arms round and round – use centrifugal force to push blood and warmth back into the fingers.

Cold sores A little ice held on the sore will often relieve the pain.

Colds and flu Colds are transmitted by direct touch. And the commonest route seems to be fingers to eyes. So don't let your children keep touching their eyes when there are bugs about.

Coughing at night This is often caused by the fact that the temperature in the bedroom is lower than in the rest of the house. Try warming the bedroom air half an hour before your child goes to bed.

Cradle cap Soften it with a little oil and then wash it away with soap and water.

Cramps Tell your child to stand barefoot and to face a wall. The wall should be about two feet away. Get him to lean forwards, keeping his heels on the floor, and touch the wall with his hands. He should then do little vertical press-ups. He should do this three times a day for a week.

Crying Try stroking the skin on his head or neck gently with one finger – moving the finger in one direction only. Do this for five minutes. If he hasn't stopped crying by then call the doctor.

Eye infection Try hot spoon bathing. Tie a piece of lint around a wooden spoon, dip it into water that has just boiled and hold it near to the affected eye. The steam that is given off will help. Do remember that conjunctivitis is very infectious. Don't let a child with an eye infection share a towel with anyone else.

Fainting Sit him down with his head between his knees. Or lie him down. Loosen clothing. Keep him in the shade. Keep him quiet.

Fever Use tepid water, not cold water, to cool your child.

Foreign body in the ear Never put anything smaller than your elbow into an ear. As long as there is no pain or history of damage or infection try pouring in a little olive oil to wash out the object.

Foreign body in the eye Fill an egg cup with boiled water containing a little salt. Get your child to hold the egg cup against his eye and to blink furiously so that the eyelid splashes in the water.

Foreign body in the nose Close the clear nostril by pressing on it with your fingers. Then tell your child to blow hard down his nose! However, don't let children with colds blow too hard – they can force germs into the middle ear!

Glue – areas of skin stuck together Don't try forcing the skin areas apart – use ordinary warm, soapy water.

Headache Is the light good enough? Poor light causes many headaches. If he gets a lot of headaches give him a couple of glasses of water a day.

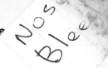

Hiccups Get your child to swallow a teas⌐

Indigestion Try getting your child⌐   ⌐de if the indigestion only affects him at ni⌐

Nappy rash Let him crawl⌐

Nose bleed Squeeze⌐   nose for ten minutes – get him to grip a l⌐   for the whole of that time. (The cork kee⌐   ⌐ps him sniffing!) Put a little petroleum je⌐   each morning and evening for a few d⌐   stop the area drying out and bleedir⌐

Ring stu⌐   ⌐ece of string around the finger on the fingertip side⌐   ⌐t fairly tightly and as close to the ring as you can get. Wi⌐   ⌐d the string you'll find that the ring will move a little way al⌐   ⌐inger. Now wind the string around the next bit of finger. And slow⌐ ⌐iove the ring towards the finger tip.

Sleeplessness Try using the vacuum cleaner if your baby can't get to sleep. Some babies seem to find the rhythmic sound of the cleaner hypnotic.

Sore throat Gargling with a teaspoonful of salt in a glass of water is the quickest way to tackle a sore throat.

Splinters Anaesthetise the area with a piece of ice – just hold the ice against the area until the skin becomes numb. Then use a sterilised needle to get the splinter out.

Sprains Try an old-fashioned compress – fold a piece of gauze, lint or other material and soak it in cold water. Then bandage it in place.

Stings If it's a bee sting you need to tease it out sideways with a sterile needle. The pain of any sting can be relieved by using a lump of ice or a little sodium bicarbonate solution. Or try soluble aspirin. Incidentally, if you're trying to sterilise a needle fix it first into a bottle cork. Then you can hold it in the flame.

Teething Dab a little alcohol on to the affected gum – it sometimes helps.

Wind Sit him up or stand him up! You don't necessarily have to pat him on the back.

Worms Children with worms have usually caught them from a dog. And a child with an itchy bottom has got worms until proved otherwise. The answer? Ask your pharmacist to recommend a product containing a worm killer.

Keeping your child healthy

Everything you need to know about feeding your child

The truth about breast feeding

1 The breasts consist of milk glands which grow during pregnancy under hormonal influence. As a result both the breasts and the nipples increase in size. Some secretion of breast milk starts towards the end of the pregnancy but it is only when the baby starts sucking at the breast that the production of milk becomes continuous.

2 Once breast feeding has become established a mother will start producing milk at the slightest stimulus. Many mothers produce milk if they just think about their baby.

3 In the first few days after birth a special type of breast milk called colostrum is produced. Colostrum is very rich in all the basic body-building ingredients that a baby needs. It is also rich in the antibodies which provide the newborn baby with protection against infection.

4 Human milk is quite different to other types of milk. It contains a unique mixture of water, protein, fat, lactose, minerals and vitamins. It is specifically formulated for human babies.

5 In order to produce a good supply of milk nursing mothers need to eat well both during and after pregnancy. There is evidence that women who do best at breast feeding will usually increase their calorie intake during their milk-producing weeks by something like 40 per cent.

6 To prepare the breasts for breast feeding the mother-to-be should pull and stretch her nipples about a dozen times every day. By pulling on the skin around the nipples it is possible to prevent the nipples becoming sore. It is also possible to increase the size of small nipples this way.

7 To prevent engorgement of one breast it is vital to make sure that the baby feeds from each breast in turn.

8 The nipples should be washed in plain water during pregnancy and before each feed. Soapy water should not be used as it will wash away the natural oils.

9 Pre-term babies and babies born with physical deformities (e.g. cleft palates) may have difficulty in sucking. If for any reason your baby cannot take milk straight from the breast then you should try expressing your milk by hand and feeding it to your baby with a spoon. As the baby grows he may be able to start sucking at the breast directly.

10 The production of milk is stimulated by sucking. If breast feeding has stopped for any reason it can usually be restarted by allowing your baby to suck at your breasts regularly each day. Sucking stimulates milk production.

11 If your nipples are short or flat then a little gentle traction should pull them out so that they can more easily be sucked.

12 If your breasts are very enlarged you may need to keep your baby's nose free so that he can breathe easily while he feeds.

13 To begin with you should feed your baby on demand. This may mean feeding ten or even more times a day. The more you feed, the more milk you will produce. If you don't seem to be producing enough milk then don't be tempted to feed with a bottle as a supplementary source. If you use a bottle then you'll never get your breast milk production up!

14 When your baby is sucking the whole of the nipple and a part of the areola around the nipple should be in his mouth. He shouldn't be 'hanging' on to the breast by the nipple or pulling at the breast either.

15 A plastic tea strainer worn inside your bra will help keep sore nipples well protected. Sore nipples should be kept dry.

16 Change your baby's position at successive feeds so that the pressure of his gums is exerted on different parts of your nipple.

17 If one nipple is persistently sore feed your baby first from the less sore nipple. This means that by the time your baby starts sucking on the sore nipple all the appropriate reflexes will have been stimulated and the milk flow will be started.

18 Wet your nipple with a little breast milk before feeding starts – this helps prevent soreness developing.

19 If breast feeding is impossible or too painful then express your milk. You can do this by hand. Hold each breast in turn in both hands and gently squeeze it towards the nipple. As your fingers reach the nipple gradually increase the pressure and squeeze the milk out. Do this four or five times and then repeat the general massage to fill up the ducts again. Any ducts which feel lumpy need slightly more enthusiastic massage. Once milk has been expressed it can be fed to your baby on a spoon or in a cup.

20 Research teams have shown that allergy problems occur less often among babies who have been fed exclusively on breast milk than among babies fed cows' milk. One team has shown that breast fed infants have an 8 per cent chance of developing eczema, whereas bottle fed infants have a 50 per cent chance of developing eczema. Other allergy problems such as asthma also seem to be related to feeding. The best protection is provided when the baby is fed exclusively on breast milk.

21 Mothers who plan to breast feed should buy bras of a slightly larger size than usual. Front fastening bras are obviously more convenient.

22 If your breasts are too full at the start of a feed and your baby can't get started then gently express a few drops of milk to make the breasts softer.

23 If your breasts still contain milk even when your baby has had enough to drink gently express the rest to prevent your breasts becoming engorged.

24 Breast size has nothing much to do with milk production. Women with small breasts can feed their babies very successfully.

25 Babies fed at the breast stand a reduced chance of becoming obese. There are several reasons for this. First, the breast feeding mother isn't tempted to empty the container in the way that the bottle feeding mother may be tempted. Second, breast milk contents change towards the end of a feed and have a reducing effect on the baby's appetite. Third, mothers preparing bottle feeds are often tempted to 'add one for the pot'. In this case the pot appears around the baby's waist.

26 Babies fed on breast milk are less likely to develop intestinal infections than babies fed on bottle milk. The breast milk container doesn't need to be cleaned or sterilised.

27 Breast feeding reduces the chances of conception if you're living on a very frugal diet. However, if you're eating well then breast feeding does not seem to be a very effective contraceptive.

28 The milk produced by a mother of a premature infant contains an abnormally high protein content – just what the premature baby needs.

29 If you're breast feeding then don't take any over-the-counter medicine, don't take alcohol and don't eat large quantities of any particular type of food. Women who are breast feeding should not take any drugs at all (and that includes the contraceptive pill) unless the drugs are essential. Under those circumstances it might be wisest to discontinue breast feeding either permanently or temporarily.

30 The incidence of breast cancer seems to be lower among women who have breast fed. This may be due to some physiological process or it may simply be a result of the fact that women who breast feed tend to be less repressed as a group than women who don't. There is strong evidence linking certain types of personality to cancer.

31 When a woman breast feeds hormones are produced which stimulate the contraction of her womb. This means that the breast feeding woman is more likely to get a flat stomach quicker.

32 Although they may still conceive breast feeding mothers tend to have irregular periods. Many consider this an advantage.

33 It is easy for a woman who is breast feeding to develop a close relationship with her baby. She has to cuddle her child every time she feeds it.

34 A baby feeding at the breast will usually spend about twenty minutes sucking. That's ten minutes at each breast.

35 If the milk ducts become blocked a hard, painful area can develop within the breast. The blocked area can sometimes be unblocked if it is stroked towards the nipple. Alternatively, if the breast with the blocked duct is favoured when offering a nipple to the baby the blockage may release itself.

36 If a breast becomes painful and swollen then mastitis may be the cause. Some experts say that mothers with mastitis should continue to breast feed. This can, however, be extremely painful. See your doctor and talk it over with him. If the breast becomes very sore an abcess may be the cause. Again you should visit your doctor.

37 Babies being fed on the breast sometimes need extra quantities of milk when they go through a growth spurt. If your baby demands additional milk then give him an extra chance at your nipples. You'll produce more milk by letting your baby suckle at your breasts more often.

38 Because breast milk is perfectly formulated there is often little waste. If your baby has irregular stools but seems well otherwise then don't worry.

39 Although lots of women think they'll find breast feeding embarrassing few do. It isn't usually difficult to find a quiet spot in which to breast feed.

40 If you're going back to work and you intend to carry on breast feeding do remember that you may need to feed several times during the normal working day. Breast feeding can be demanding and disruptive.

41 If you cannot feed your baby exclusively on breast milk you may still be able to feed him some milk expressed from your breasts. Failing that you may even be able to obtain surplus human breast milk from a local 'milk bank.'

Bottle feeding

1 If breast milk isn't available there is much that you can do to ensure that bottle feeding is a successful alternative. It is often said that breast feeding enables mothers to build a bond with their baby. This is undoubtedly true but just because you're bottle feeding that is no reason why you shouldn't build the same sort of bond. Make sure that you hold your baby close to you when you bottle feed and *never* leave your baby alone with his bottle. (This is in any case a dangerous practice since a baby propped up with a bottle by his side can easily choke on inhaled milk.)

2 Most special baby milks start off as cows' milk. Some are offered with half the water removed (as evaporated milk) while others are offered with all the water removed (as dried milk). When choosing a suitable type of milk for bottle feeding you should take the advice of your doctor or midwife.

3 Once you've selected a brand of milk to use follow the manufacturer's instructions carefully. Do not be tempted to add extra milk powder to the preparation and don't add extra sugar, salt or vitamins. You're likely to do your baby more harm than good.

4 When feeding a baby out of a bottle it is important to sterilise the bottle carefully. Again, whatever method of sterilisation you use it is vital to follow all the instructions carefully. Do that and you'll have no problems. Try finding short cuts and you'll endanger your baby.

5 There is no evidence that by giving your baby larger than normal feeds you will increase the interval between feeds.

6 Make sure that you don't run out of the type of milk you're using. If you do run out you'll be tempted to substitute ordinary dairy milk – and that could be dangerous.

7 Even if you are not breast feeding your breasts may still be producing milk. Consult your doctor for advice. Generally speaking, however, if there is no sucking then milk production will gradually halt.

8 Bottle fed babies usually become used to a routine rather quicker than breast fed babies. It's easier to feed your baby when you want to feed him rather than when he wants to be fed. On the whole, however, I recommend that you allow your baby to determine the feeding routine. Remember that if you encourage your baby to follow his natural appetite then you're unlikely to have a fat baby or a fat child.

9 If there is milk left in the bottle and your baby seems full then don't be tempted to force him to finish off the bottle!

10 You can prepare bottle feeds and leave them in the fridge. Again make sure that you follow all the relevant instructions.

15 One important advantage with bottle feeding is that anyone can do the feeding – and mother can go to work. Do remember, however, that it is important not to leave your baby alone with his bottle. He needs cuddling when he is feeding.

Weaning and after

1 Whether you're breast feeding or bottle feeding your baby he'll happily survive on milk for between four and six months. At that age you can start weaning. Children's intestines aren't ready to deal with solids before then.

2 If you start your baby on solids too soon you'll run the risk of making him fat. And fat babies are not bonny – they're unhealthy.

3 Tins of baby food are all right but there is no reason why you shouldn't start your baby on real, healthy, wholesome food. Give your baby a raw carrot or stick of celery to chew.

4 Don't add salt or sugar to your baby's meals. You can easily produce problems if you do. And you may also start bad habits that will be difficult to stop.

5 Offer your baby a good variety of natural foods. But if he doesn't like something don't get involved in any major battles at this stage.

6 Don't give your baby or toddler sweets between meals. If you do you'll be starting a bad habit that will be difficult to stop. Babies aren't born with a 'sweet tooth' – they acquire it because parents and kindly relatives keep giving them sweets.

7 Most babies can start using spoons and cups at about six months of age. But don't worry if he makes a mess!

8 Babies and young children are very capable of deciding for themselves exactly what they need to eat. Your child may seem to be eating an odd diet but unless he isn't thriving or seems ill you needn't worry.

9 You don't need to add extra vitamins or minerals to your child's diet if he is eating a normal, varied selection of foodstuffs. Too many vitamins can be as dangerous as too few vitamins.

10 If you want to start your child on a vegetarian or vegan diet (or any other special diet) do please seek professional advice first. A report in the *British Medical Journal* in 1979 pointed out that children have become dangerously ill after having been put on vegetarian and macrobiotic diets. This sort of infant feeding has been designated a form of child abuse.

11 The baby who has recurrent colic, vomiting, diarrhoea or constipation is probably being overfed. The baby who fails to gain enough weight, who draws up his legs in discomfort or who has difficulty in getting off to sleep is probably being underfed.

12 When older children get constipated you should try changing their diet a little. Add more fresh fruit, more green vegetables, more fluids and less starchy foods. If that doesn't work try adding a little bran to the morning breakfast cereal.

See also
Anorexia, page 25.
Appetite loss, page 30.
Food allergy, page 138.
Obesity, page 190.
Wind, page 251.

Looking after your child's teeth

Dental decay is one of the commonest diseases in the western world, producing pain, poor eating habits and much distress and embarrassment. It is now quite well established that dietary habits are largely responsible for this epidemic of dental decay. Medical historians have carefully traced the increase in dental decay back to the seventeenth century when people in Britain first began to eat sugar in relatively large quantities. More recently added evidence has been obtained from the fact that tooth decay among the Eskimos has risen as they have adopted the American junk diet with its heavy sugar content.

There is much that you can do to help your child preserve his teeth by encouraging him to chew sugar-free foods. If you encourage your child to nibble fresh fruit and washed raw vegetables you'll help in two main ways. First, the chewing will help clean the teeth in a purely mechanical fashion and the production of large quantities of saliva will help too. Second, you'll be helping to prevent your child getting a harmful taste for sweet foods. While on the subject of foods, by the way, it is worth remembering that milk is an excellent source of calcium and phosphorus, both of which are needed by developing teeth.

To fluoride or not to fluoride
During the last few years there has been a huge public controversy over the importance of fluoride in the protection of teeth. It was back in 1892 that it was first suggested that the high incidence of dental caries or tooth decay in England might be due to a deficiency of fluoride in the diet. Tooth enamel contains a substance called hydroxyapatite which, with the addition of fluoride, is converted to a much harder and decay-resistant substance called fluorpatite.

When it became clear that in those geographical regions where the water supply contains enough natural fluoride the incidence of tooth decay is low a number of scientists suggested adding fluoride to drinking water supplies. Not unnaturally this suggestion produced a great deal of controversy and stimulated much heated discussion. It was pointed out that adding fluoride to the drinking water could well be just the sharp end of a rather large wedge.

To a large extent, however, the arguments that have taken place have been unnecessary since it is relatively simple to provide fluoride protection at home. A three-year study conducted in schools in seventeen American communities that did not have fluoride in the water showed that a weekly fluoride mouthwash programme is an easy, cheap and effective way to reduce decay. Fluoride toothpaste can do the same job as a mouthwash.

Teeth cleaning habits

You can do a lot to help your children grow up with strong healthy teeth by teaching him good teeth cleaning habits early in life. Proper teeth cleaning habits need to be continued regularly if teeth are to be protected against the sticky, colourless film which is made up of a mixture of saliva, food debris and bacteria and which is known as plaque. When sugary substances come into contact with the bacteria found in plaque they form acids which start the decaying process.

Clearing away the plaque is obviously an important part of tooth hygiene. The first problem, however, is that the plaque is invisible. You can get over this hurdle by buying special 'disclosing tablets'. When chewed these tablets leave a pink or blue stain on the teeth which will remain until the plaque has been properly removed.

Your child will need three other weapons in his fight against plaque. These are:

1 A good toothbrush Buy a brush with bristles that feel soft to the touch. It doesn't matter whether the bristles are nylon or natural. Nor does it matter much whether the ends of the individual bristles are rounded. Buy a brush with a flat head, not one with a contoured head or a head with different lengths of bristle.

When the old brush is worn and the bristles are bent buy a new one. Press the bristles down with your finger to test them. If they don't spring back into position then the brush should be retired to cleaning typewriter keys. Most people need a new brush every three months.

Electric toothbrushes are useful for children who are disabled or have difficulty in holding an ordinary toothbrush for any reason.

2 A toothpaste Traditionally toothpastes worked because in addition to containing flavouring and a detergent they included an abrasive which helped to scrub the plaque away. If your child uses too abrasive a paste or powder, however, he may actually wear away the surface of his teeth (and leave them sensitive to particularly cold or sweet products). I suggest that you avoid powders which tend to be particularly abrasive.

The major step forward in the world of toothpaste manufacture has involved the addition of fluoride. There is certainly good evidence to show that the child who uses a toothpaste containing fluoride will be better protected against tooth decay than a child using any other type of paste.

3 Dental floss Dental floss is simply a thin thread which can be used to reach between the teeth. It is important to be gentle when using floss. If used carelessly floss can cut into the gums like a cheesewire into a ripe Camembert. Using floss is very easy. All your child has to do is break off a length of the thin cotton-like substance (waxed or unwaxed – it doesn't really matter) and wind both ends round the fingers of his two hands. Then he inserts the taut strand between two teeth and pulls it up and down to clean away the plaque.

There are all sorts of other teeth cleaning products available. You can, for example, buy battery-operated tooth polishers and forced irrigation devices (designed to clean your teeth by squirting jets of water on to and between them) but I don't think you need buy anything else at all. Antiseptic mouthwashes and rinses are, in my view, a complete waste of time and money.

What you do need to remember is that the teeth need to be cleaned regularly and well. Cleaning the teeth will probably take three or four minutes if done properly. One good clean done every evening will be more useful than several half-hearted attempts during the daytime.

Looking after your child's feet

Most children start off with well-shaped, flawless feet. The problems which frequently develop and which can cause so much discomfort in later life are often due to poor foot care in childhood.

Good foot care needs to begin shortly after birth.

The good foot guide
1 Shoes, socks or stretch suits that do not leave room for growth or movement can do a great deal of damage to growing feet. It is

forgotten that socks and stretch suits that aren't really big enough can prove dangerously restrictive.

2 Babies don't need to wear shoes until they're walking around by themselves. Until then they should be allowed to remain barefoot.

3 Always buy shoes from a shop where the assistants have the time and knowledge to measure your child's feet properly. Good shoes are made in several widths and fittings to each half size. Both feet should be measured every time shoes are bought and they should be measured with your child standing up straight.

4 Make sure that the shoes you buy are big enough. There should be three quarters of an inch between the tip of the longest toe and the front of the shoe. A quick way to check that a shoe is big enough is to ask your child to push his toes right to the front of the shoe. You should then be able to get your finger between the back of your child's heel and the back of the shoe. Encourage your child to try on both shoes and walk about in them.

5 If it is at all possible buy shoes in the afternoon rather than the morning. Feet are bigger later on in the day.

6 Don't buy stacked heels, high heels or pointed toe shoes except for 'fun wear' at parties. Everyday shoes need to be comfortable and well-fitting.

7 Children shouldn't have Sunday Best shoes. If shoes are kept for special occasions they will be too small long before they have been worn out. It pays to buy one pair of good shoes, look after them and replace them when they are worn out or too small.

8 Shoes that have laces or adjustable straps are best. They hold the foot firmly in position even though there may be space available.

9 When you're buying new shoes check that they are firm but supple. Shoes need to provide support but should also bend with the foot.

10 Pumps, trainers and plimsolls are not sensible shoes for regular wear. They are rarely available in a full range of sizes and they often make the feet sweat. They should be kept for occasional, leisure and sports wear.

11 Rubber and synthetic shoes tend to make sweating worse. Leather shoes are usually the best buy in the long run.

12 Socks and stockings should be changed and washed daily whenever possible.

13 The feet should be washed daily but should also be dried carefully afterwards. The area between the toes is often left damp. This can easily lead to the growth of fungal infections. It's much easier to contract foot infections than it is to get rid of them.

14 If your child tends to suffer from dry, cracked skin on his feet put an ordinary moisturising cream on after washing.

15 Toenail care is important. Teach your child to use a nailbrush to remove ingrained dirt and loose, dead, surface skin cells. Toenails should be cut straight across to avoid the development of ingrowing toenails.

Don't put your child under too much pressure

Children are just as susceptible to pressure and stress as adults. Something like one half of all childhood illnesses and ailments are either produced or exacerbated by stress. Follow the advice below to avoid putting your child under too much stress.

Don't manipulate your child

As parents we are skilled at getting our children to do what we want them to do by making them feel guilty. When you say 'you wouldn't do that if you loved me', 'if you only knew what sacrifices we've made for you', 'you're making your mother ill' or 'I don't know what we've done to deserve this sort of treatment' you are manipulating your child by using guilt as a weapon. You may not be consciously attempting to force your child to behave in a particular way but unconsciously you're doing just that. Guilt is an extremely powerful weapon and is particularly dangerous when allowed to intrude into a relationship based largely on love and affection.

The more sensitive your child is the more likely he is to be put under pressure and stress by such simple manipulative phrases. And gentle, emotional blackmail of this kind produces more long-lasting and damaging stress than shouting, screaming, threatening or even beating your child!

Don't put your child under too much pressure to succeed

We live in a very competitive society and today children of all ages are encouraged to do well in many different ways. By the time they reach the age of 6 or 7 years children are already under pressure to do well to school.

There are even many parents and teachers who put their children under pressure to do well on the sports fields and in the athletics arena. There are cups to be won, prizes to be collected and trophies to be accumulated. I've seen toddlers crying because their team has been beaten and I've met children with hands blistered by hours of practice with the tennis racket or golf club.

Don't put too much pressure on your child to grow up

A remarkable number of children who are struggling to cope with the physical, mental and emotional problems of puberty are also expected to cope with some of the responsibilities normally shouldered by adults.

I've met children who have been expected to do the family shopping and housework, children who have been making their own meals at the age of 10 and children who've been expected to act as interpreters and translators for entire families. Often children with one parent will be expected to provide support, advice and comfort in place of the missing spouse.

Try to let your child enjoy his childhood. He won't get another chance.

Protect him from the advertisers

Children adapt to change very well these days. Even quite small children quickly become accustomed to the fact that there are few stable factors in the world around them. Buildings are knocked down, pop singers go in and out of fashion, clothes that are 'with it' one month can be unwearable a few weeks later.

Nevertheless, there are some aspects of modern life that even children may find daunting. By the time he is old enough to vote your child will have watched something like 100,000 television commercials, seen thousands of newspaper and magazine advertisements and been exposed to advertising propaganda while in the cinemas and while listening to the radio.

It is hardly surprising that, under these continuing pressures, many children grow up with entirely artificial tastes and needs; tastes and needs that have been designed and nurtured by an unseen army of hidden manipulators.

You may be able to help your child cope with this deluge of commercially inspired misinformation by teaching him a little scepticism and cynicism!

The bogey man lives – but in Hollywood

The television set is commonly used as a permanently available electronic babysitter. Children love the 'box' so much that when a group of 4- to 6-year-olds were recently asked which they liked best, television or daddy, nearly half said that they preferred TV.

And yet it is now a recognised fact that many children have nightmares as a direct result of watching frightening films on television. A recent survey showed that one in three school children dream about programmes they have watched. When you realise that a TV diet consists largely of murders, butchery and rape it is hardly surprising that children's viewing habits often lead to nightmares.

Just as the variety of pressures likely to affect children is great so there are a large number of different symptoms known to be stress-related in children. You should always think of stress as a possible cause if your child complains of vague symptoms such as lethargy and general tiredness but there are also some specific physical problems which are well known to be produced by stress.

Here are some of the commonest stress-related disorders:

1 Abdominal pain Although appendicitis is very common it isn't as common a cause of abdominal pain in children as anxiety. Between a third and a half of all the appendices removed are, in fact, perfectly healthy! Stress-induced abdominal pains can usually be clearly related to a particular type of pressure. Pains which come on a Monday morning and which go by midday are often produced by fears associated with school. (See page 7.)

2 Accidents More children die of accidents than die of pneumonia, heart disease, cancer and meningitis. Among all children over the age of 1 year accidents are the commonest cause of death and serious injury.

And yet accidents aren't usually accidental. Most are caused by something. And that something is often stress. The child who is anxious and under pressure will not be able to concentrate properly on what is going on. He'll be accident-prone. So, if your child is permanently decorated with grubby bits of sticking plaster then you should perhaps ask yourself whether he could be worrying about problems at home or at school. (See page 12.)

3 Appetite loss Children under pressure often lose their appetites (see page 30). Sometimes the loss of appetite can produce a frightening weight loss. Anorexia nervosa, a condition in which children more or less stop eating altogether, is discussed on page 25.

4 Asthma Asthma is a condition that is often very obviously made worse by stress. Parents who openly row with one another or who put a great deal of pressure on their children may well find that none of the usually effective anti-asthma drugs do any good. At the other end of the scale parents who make too much fuss may make asthma worse. (See page 33.)

5 Bedwetting The child who wets his bed regularly may be a regular worrier too. When children continue to wet their beds after the age of 5 or 6 years and there is no known physical cause then stress may well be behind it. The more pressure parents put on a child not to wet his bed the more likely the problem is to continue. (See page 40.)

6 Eczema When we're frightened we go white. When we're angry we go red. When we're embarrassed we blush. When we're anxious we sweat.

The skin is pretty obviously affected by feelings and emotions of all kinds. And stress can produce eczema or make an existing patch of eczema worse. (See page 120.)

7 Headaches All sorts of headaches – ranging from the simple headache across the front of the head to the full-blooded migraine headache – can be produced or made worse by stress and tension. If your child gets lots of headaches then it may be that he's pushing himself too hard. Or you're pushing him too hard. Either way he may benefit by learning how to relax properly. (See page 152.)

8 Nail biting You may be able to stop nail biting by painting your child's nails with a foul-tasting varnish or by encouraging him to take pride in the appearance of his nails but it is important to remember that children who are always nibbling at their nails usually do so because they are anxious.

Find out why your child is anxious and you may be able to stop the nail biting at source!

9 Sleeplessness Children often lie awake because they are anxious about relationships at home or about problems at school. They also fail to get to sleep because they've been frightened by a scary TV film. (See pages 188 and 213.)

10 Thumb sucking Children usually 'kick' the thumb sucking habit by the time they reach the age of 3 or 4. When they don't then it may be because of stress. (See page 143.)

11 Tics and twitches Winking, blinking, coughing, sighing and many other unexpected, rapid, involuntary repetitive movements which seem to serve no purpose at all are often a result of stress and tension. (See page 230.)

Protect your child against stress

1 You must understand what sort of things can produce stress. If you push your child too hard, if you expect too much or if you give him too much responsibility then you might be adding to his stress. Some of the commoner causes of stress among children are described on page 288.

2 You should look for early signs of stress. If your child suffers from any of the problems listed above then you should always think of stress as a possible cause. Children who seem to get upset very easily are also likely to be suffering from stress.

3 Don't always expect your child to be doing something useful. Many parents tell their children off if they find them daydreaming but in fact daydreaming is a simple and very natural way of relaxing. There is nothing wrong with your child escaping from the real world into a daydream every now and again! The only time to get worried is if he doesn't seem to be coming back to reality.

4 Don't let your child get involved in too many high pressure activities. Encourage him to spend some time at least relaxing on things that don't really matter very much.

5 Do try and spend some time each day talking to your child, finding out what sort of things are worrying him and encouraging him to share his problems with you.

Bad habits

When they think of drug dependence and addiction problems most parents think of heroin, morphine, cocaine and the hard drugs. Dangerous as these drugs are, however, there are other far more common problems to be aware of. The number of children and youngsters who die each year after abusing alcohol, taking prescribed drugs and sniffing glue and other solvents far exceeds the number who die after using hard drugs. The chances are high that one or more of the children your child meets daily will be a regular user of some toxic and potentially dangerous substance.

There is no certain way to ensure that your child never becomes habituated or addicted. But you can reduce the risks.
1 Talk to your child and let him grow up accustomed to the idea that he can discuss problems, fears, worries and dilemmas openly with you.
2 Discuss the reasons why people take drugs, what the advantages may be and what the disadvantages are.
3 Children under stress are more likely to turn to drugs for support than other youngsters. Try not to put your child under too much pressure. Be on the look-out for early warning signs of excessive pressure.

If despite your efforts you notice that your child is behaving abnormally in any way, if he starts to lose weight, if he begins to complain of inexplicable physical symptoms or if he is always short of money then don't refuse to accept the possibility that he may be using some sort of drugs. The sooner you seek professional help the better the chances of finding the solution you want.

Keeping your child healthy: quick tips

If first aid is needed and you're not certain about what to do – do nothing.

If your daughter has her ears pierced make sure that it is done by someone who uses sterile equipment. The ears shouldn't be pierced if there is any infection present. Sterling silver rings or gold of 14 carats or more are least likely to cause problems.

Swimming baths are often rich in chlorine – protect your child's eyes by giving him goggles to wear.

Salt is an excellent emergency antiseptic. If your child cuts or grazes himself then put a pinch of salt in his next few baths. It will help prevent infection developing.

Don't let children travel in tight clothing. If you do they'll get cramp.

Children with itchy rashes often scratch at night. And that can cause infection. So get your child to wear gloves or mittens at night if you think he's likely to end up scratching.

Don't let children with colds blow up balloons – the high pressure can push germs into the middle ear.

Don't let young sportsmen use pain-relieving sprays – they can mask injuries and result in minor problems becoming major problems.

Remember the five day rule – if it isn't better in five days then you need medical advice.

Children who are regular targets for biting insects may get protection if they take vitamin B – the vitamin is excreted in the sweat and it makes the skin taste funny. Remember too that yellow clothes attract insects.

Every night hundreds of teenage girls have sex for the first time. Less than half use any form of contraception.

In cold weather it is better to keep a child's bedroom warm than to pile more and more clothes on to the bed.

Small boys sometimes use rubber bands to hold their socks up. These home made garters are potentially dangerous – they cut off the circulation.

Don't let small children play in the sun for more than a few minutes at a time. Remember that floppy hats, loose-fitting clothes and tons of moisturising cream will provide much-needed protection.

Don't let small children wander around on rocky or pebbly beaches barefoot. They'll be much safer in last year's shoes with the toes cut out. Let them go into the sea in them too.

Teach your child to lift properly and you'll protect him from backache. Lifting should be done with the back straight and the legs bent.

Let your child cry if he wants to. It is dangerous to suppress emotions. Even boys should be allowed to cry when they need to.

If you smoke don't smoke in the room where your child spends much time. Children of heavy-smoking parents are more likely to get chest infections, ear infections and sore throats than other children.

If you're burning rubbish on your garden bonfire keep children away. Apart from the danger of their being burnt there is another risk – household items often contain chemicals which give off dangerous fumes when burnt.

If anyone in your home has a serious infection sterilise plates and cutlery by using ordinary domestic bleach. Wash in bleach and then clean thoroughly in ordinary soapy water. Then rinse.

If you're travelling by car don't let children sit on your lap in the front seat. Don't let them lean out of the window. And don't let them stand up. They should be fastened in with seat belts wherever they are sitting. Make sure your car has rear doors which lock. And lock them! If you're planning a long journey pack some rugs and cushions so that children can sleep. And pack flasks of cold drinks and moist tissues too.

Children up to 7 need about fourteen hours sleep. Children of 8 to 12 need eleven to twelve hours. Between 12 and 16 nine to eleven hours is average.

Although children like sticking plasters (as badges of merit and bravery), most small cuts and grazes get better quicker if left to heal in the open air. Wash well with a liquid antiseptic and water.

If you're going shopping in a crowded store always arrange to meet your child at some specific point should you get parted.

Never give a child with abdominal pain anything by mouth. Wipe his face and lips with a damp cloth. At most let him suck a small piece of ice.

Don't leave old fridges, car batteries or other pieces of potentially dangerous junk lying around the garden.

Don't let your child kiss a pet. And make sure he washes his hands after playing with a pet. Many infections that are harmless to animals can affect children.

If your child has a long-term illness encourage him to learn as much about it as possible.

If your child has a long-term problem (such as diabetes, epilepsy or an allergy) but him a necklace or bracelet on which information about his medical condition can be engraved. Your doctor or pharmacist will have details of suitable devices.

Professional help

As far as you and your child are concerned the most important doctor in your life should be your family doctor or general practitioner. Medicine is a complex, sophisticated business and even in the apparently specialised world of paediatrics there are dozens of subspecialities. There are paediatricians specialising in psychiatric problems, in chest surgery, in hormonal problems and in the whole range of medical and surgical disorders. To make sure that your child receives the correct help from the correct specialist you must have access to a family doctor who will retain overall control of your child's health but be prepared to make referrals as and when they are needed.

Choosing a doctor

You need to know that your doctor is properly qualified. It is illegal for anyone who does not have acceptable medical qualifications to claim to be a fully registered medical practitioner. All registered medical practitioners will be listed in the official directories and registers which can usually be found in local libraries. Look up any doctors you're planning to consult and check that they are properly qualified. Do not, however, be overimpressed by a string of qualifications. A good academic doctor isn't necessarily a good clinician or a good family doctor.

You'll want to look at the way that the practice is run, too, before you consider joining a doctor. A few telephone calls should quickly tell you everything you need to know. You'll want to know whether a doctor runs an appointment system or simply sees patients when they turn up. You'll want to know whether the doctor is in single-handed practice or a member of a partnership and you may want to investigate the sex, age or nationality of the doctors concerned. The structure of the practice you're going to join is undoubtedly important but don't be overawed by an impressive office layout. The vast variety of statistics which exist in medical libraries around the world show that there is no steady relationship between the way in which a practice is structured and the quality or effectiveness of the care provided.

It will be important too to choose a practice that isn't too far away from your home. There is little point in joining a practice with a marvellous doctor in attendance if you have to spend eight hours sitting on buses every time you want to obtain advice. If you live in a country area you'll probably not have much choice but if you live in a city or large town then you'll probably have the choice of half a dozen doctors or even more.

Finally, before you start visiting a doctor talk to a few friends and neighbours. Be careful not to take advice from only one acquaintance – you may be listening to someone with a grudge or someone who is easily impressed. By talking to two or three people, however, it should be possible to acquire a reliable impression and decide whether the practitioner you are considering offers impersonal efficiency, friendly chaos or an acceptable mixture of both.

Getting the best out of your doctor

1 Stick with him if you can. It takes time to build up a good doctor-patient relationship. If you find a good doctor whom you trust then treat him with care and affection. If you find a good doctor whom you trust but who has a few flaws decide whether or not you think you can do better elsewhere. If you can't, and you can put up with the flaws, then do the best you can to keep the relationship smooth.

2 Most children can safely be moved to the doctor's consulting room even when they are ill. Small children, in particular, can usually be wrapped up and transported to the consulting room. Doctors prefer patients to come to them partly because it saves time but also because they know that they will have access to the instruments and equipment they may need. Ask for a home visit only if you feel that you cannot move your child without adding to his discomfort or making his condition worse.

3 If you need emergency help then do make the nature of the emergency clear to the receptionist or whoever it is you speak to and do make sure that the doctor is told where the child is. Valuable time will be wasted if your doctor visits your home address while your child is staying with grandparents across town.

4 When booking a routine appointment make it clear just what you need. If you are taking your child along for a routine vaccination you may be booked into a special immunisation clinic. If you need a full medical examination extra appointment time may need to be allocated.

5 Don't book an appointment for one child and then ask for advice about half a dozen other children, a couple of stray aunties and your grandfather. You'll annoy your doctor and the people waiting to see him and you'll probably get inadequate answers because the medical records may not be immediately available.

6 Think about what you want to tell the doctor – and what you expect from the doctor. Do not be frightened to make notes beforehand and to add to them during the consultation. Doctors write down the information that you give them and there is absolutely no reason why you shouldn't jot down what you get in return. Tell the doctor:

(a) all the symptoms that you have noticed – even if they don't seem entirely relevant to you. If you have dates – so much the better.

(b) details of any remedies you've tried.

(c) any family history or past medical events that might be significant.

(d) about any recent trips that your child has made – particularly if they took him abroad.

In return you'll want to know:

(a) what he thinks is wrong. Remember, however, that not all consultations end in a diagnosis being made.

(b) whether any tests or investigations need to be done and if so when and where you have to take your child.

(c) what treatment is recommended and whether any other advice needs to be followed.

(d) whether you need to make another appointment.

Seeing a specialist

If your family doctor thinks that your child needs to be seen by a specialist he will make the appropriate referral. If you aren't happy with the way things are going and you want to have a second or specialist opinion then you should ask your doctor to make the appropriate arrangements.

When you see the specialist tell him about anything that has happened since your child was seen by your family doctor. Prepare for the specialist consultation in just the same way that you prepare for a consultation with your family doctor – make sure that you know what questions you want to ask.

After you've seen the specialist wait a few days and then make an appointment to see your own family doctor (unless the problem was a simple, straightforward one which was dealt with at the specialist consultation). Your family doctor will be able to interpret for you anything the specialist may have told you and by this time he will have probably have had a letter telling him the specialist's professional opinion.

It is important to remember that when you see a consultant your doctor is not handing over care of your child but asking for help and advice. If you are to get the best out of your relationship with your family doctor then you must make sure that he is allowed to keep overall control of your child's health.

Finally, if your own family doctor refuses to provide you with a second opinion then I suggest that you change doctors.

The alternative professionals

A growing number of patients are becoming disillusioned with orthodox medicine and are seeking help from the so-called 'alternative professionals'.

It is important to remember, however, that although the problems associated with the alternative professionals may be different there are undoubtedly just as many difficulties associated with unorthodox medical treatments as there are with the orthodox, established medical practices.

Alternative forms of medical treatment are not automatically devoid of medical risk. The dangers may be different from those associated ith surgery or modern drug therapy but they are without doubt just as real. In addition, although there is much anecdotal support for specific forms of alternative treatment there is often very little solid scientific evidence to show that the remedies offered do any good.

It is worth remembering, too, that while there are careful cautious, experienced and honourable, practitioners in the world of alternative medicine there are also flamboyant, dangerous and unqualified and unscrupulous practitioners around. Unfortunately, you as a consumer have no way of differentiating between the good, the bad and the entirely indifferent. A truly incompetent medical practitioner will lose his licence to practise. A truly incompetent unorthodox practitioner cannot be banned or removed from any register because the chances are high that he was never on one in the first place.

Using prescribed drugs safely and effectively

1 Make sure that you understand why your child has been given a drug to take. If you are worried or confused about anything relating to the drug then you should ask for advice.
2 Find out just how long the drug needs to be taken for and in precisely what dosage. Some drugs can be stopped when symptoms cease. Others need to be taken as a complete course. A few drugs need to be taken continuously and prescriptions will have to be renewed before the supply of drugs runs out. You should know what the drug is for and wht the effect will be.
3 Ask your doctor how often the drug needs to be taken. If a drug needs to be taken once a day it does not usually matter what time of day it is taken as long as it is taken at the same time each day. If a drug has to be taken twice a day then it should be taken at intervals of twelve hours. A drug that needs taking three times a day should be taken at eight-hour intervals and a drug that needs taking four times a day should be taken at six-hour intervals. The day should be divided into suitable segments.
4 Make sure you know whether the drug needs to be taken before meals, with meals or after meals. Some drugs which may cause stomach problems are safer when taken with meals. Other drugs may not be absorbed properly if taken with food. Taking pills at the wrong time can devalue their effectiveness.
5 All medicines should normally be stored in the containers in which they were supplied. The labels should not be removed and containers should be kept tightly fastened. Drugs need to be kept out of extremes of heat and cold. Drugs should, of course, be

kept in a lockable medicine cabinet.

6 If your child is taking two or more different drugs and you think you or he might get confused then make a simple daily chart to help you keep track of which pills have been given and which have not. Some people find that it helps to keep each day's medication in a separate bottle. If you do this make sure that you only move one day's supply at a time.

7 Remember that any drug that can have a useful effect on the human body can also have a damaging effect. There is no such thing as a completely safe but effective drug. Use drugs with caution and respect.

8 Teach your child to regard drugs with respect rather than fear. Do not allow your child to play with tablets or pills. On the other hand you should not forbid a child to see tablets, pills or capsules. If you make too much of a mystery out of tablets you'll encourage hazardous experimentation.

9 If your child is fit enough to go to school but needs to take tablets or medicine while there have a word with the school teacher. Explain what dose of medicine has to be taken at what time.

10 Many tablets are also available in liquid form and many liquid medicines are also available in tablet or capsule form. If your child is given a medicine in one form but prefers another form ask your doctor to make the change before the treatment starts.

11 If your child needs to take pills regularly teach him to look after his own medication as soon as you can. Diabetic children should be taught to give themselves their own injections as early as possible if they are to enjoy full independence as they grow up.

12 Don't let your child swallow pills without water. If swallowed in this way pills may stick in the gullet and cause damage. Pills should always be taken with a glass of water or wrapped up in a small pellet of bread.

13 When children are small all pills need to be kept locked up. As children grow up, however, it is wise to remove some of the mystery. Explain to them that drugs are powerful and can be dangerous if used improperly. Explain what good they can do, too.

14 If you're going abroad do make sure that you take any pills that your child needs to take. And take too a small holiday drug cabinet – take calamine for itchy rashes, kaolin for diarrhoea, antacid for stomach upsets and aspirin or paracetamol for pain.

15 If you have difficulty in persuading your baby to take medicine from a spoon then put the medicine into a teat and let your baby suck the medicine out.

16 When he's swallowing tablets get your child to hold his head back after taking a sip of water. To swallow capsules get him to hold his head forward after taking a sip. Tablets are heavy and will fall by gravity. But capsules are light and will float down the throat on a little water.

17 When small children cannot (or will not) swallow tablets it is sometimes possible to hide the tablet in a spoonful of jam or some other favourite delicacy. However, do remember that tablets should not be crushed and capsules should not be opened.

18 If a liquid medicine has been prescribed then do make sure that you shake the bottle before pouring out the recommended dose since some liquid preparations may separate during storage. Small children who refuse to take medicine can be encouraged to co-operate if you hold your child's nose gently but firmly shut and then slip the spoonful of medicine into his mouth. The swallowing reflex will do the rest.

19 Side effects with powerful drugs are, I'm afraid, common. The following list of side effects details only the commoner problems and is not intended to be comprehensive:

Constipation: Common with pain relievers, antacids, cough medicines and, naturally enough, drugs used in the treatment of diarrhoea.

Diarrhoea: Anti-infectives (such as types of penicillin) are often associated with diarrhoea as are drugs used in the treatment of gastrointestinal problems such as indigestion, gastritis and constipation.

Dizziness: Aspirin and quinine are two drugs commonly and specifically associated with dizziness. Anti-infectives and drugs used in the treatment of nerve disorders (such as anxiety and depression) are also common culprits.

Drowsiness: This is a common problem with all drugs which have an effect on the central nervous system – these include sedatives, tranquillizers, hypnotics, all drugs used in the treatment of anxiety and depression and drugs used in the treatment of epilepsy. Drowsiness is also common with antihistamines – the group of drugs used in the treatment of a wide range of allergy problems. Patients taking medication for hay fever should, for example, beware of this problem.

Dry mouth: Drugs used in the treatment of nervous problems can produce a dry mouth. So can a number of other products.

Headache: Headache is a symptom that has been associated with an enormous range of drugs. It is, however, important to remember that anxiety and tension are also common causes of headache and that a child ill enough to need medication may already be anxious or tense.

Indigestion or wind: Obviously drugs that are taken by mouth are most likely to be associated with indigestion and wind. Pain relievers, anti-infectives and steroids are particularly likely to cause these symptoms.

Itching: Itching associated with a skin rash means that an allergy reaction is almost certain.

Nausea and vomiting: A very wide range of drugs can cause nausea and sickness. Hormones, heart drugs, pain relievers and anti-infectives are four of the common groups associated with these side effects.

Skin rash: Any drug can cause this side effect. Anti-infectives, such as penicillin and sulphonamide, are perhaps most commonly associated with the problem. A skin rash usually suggests an allergy to the drug.

Other effects: Other effects which may be noticed include confusion, hallucination, tremors, fainting, wheezing, palpitations, blurred vision, depression, sweating and ringing in the ears.

If you think your child could have a drug-induced side effect then you should telephone and ask your doctor for advice if the problem is troublesome or persistent. Mildly irritating side effects can usually be safely ignored. Incidentally, if your child has a clear allergy reaction to a drug then you should make sure that your doctor makes a note of the drug responsible. You, too, should keep a record of any drug-related allergies (there is a Record Sheet on page 316 of this book). It may also be sensible to invest in a Medic Alert bracelet.

20 Do remember that drugs don't always mix well together and may, indeed, react together in a dangerous way. If your child is already taking a prescribed drug and you are offered another drug or prescription then make sure that the two products will not interact badly.

21 Prescribed drugs do not always mix well with drugs bought 'over the counter'. As a general rule you should never give your child a proprietary medicine if he is taking a prescribed medicine.

22 Do not allow your child to stop taking a drug if you have been advised to make sure he takes a full course. Ring your doctor for advice if you do need to stop for any reason. Some drugs have to be stopped gradually rather than abruptly.

23 Never give your child drugs that have been prescribed for someone else.

24 The warnings and advice given above are not intended to stop you taking advantage of the effectiveness of many modern drugs. Doctors sometimes divide patients into two groups: those who are willing to take drugs for any little symptom and those who are unwilling to take drugs under any circumstances. Try not to fall into either of these extremist groups.

Vaccines and vaccinations

If a child catches measles when he is small he will probably develop immunity. He won't catch measles again however many more times he is exposed to the infection. His body will have prepared its own defence mechanism so that any exposure to the same threatening organism will be repulsed.

The theory of vaccination is based on the fact that the human body can prepare the necessary defence mechanism without the individual actually contracting the disease. The body develops immunological defences because the vaccine provides a sneak preview of the disease concerned.

The effectiveness of different vaccines varies a good deal. For some diseases, such as polio and tetanus, the available vaccines are effective and long-lasting. For other diseases, such as cholera, vaccines are not so effective nor so long-lasting.

The risk of side effects varies too and those risks must always be weighed against the benefits. In recent years the particular vaccine which has aroused most controversy has been the one used to protect against whooping cough (pertussis). A number of expert still claim that whooping cough vaccination is not only relatively inefficient but is also responsible for a relatively high number of problems. They say that there are, in particular, unacceptable risks of brain damage. Other experts, however, claim that the risks to the community of stopping whooping cough vaccination are greater than the risks of continuing. They argue that if no babies were vaccinated against whooping cough the incidence of the disease in the community would rise alarmingly.

Nevertheless, despite these reassurances a large number of parents have in recent years chosen not to have their babies vaccinated against whooping cough. Unhappily the use of other, safer vaccines has also suffered and some young children are now unprotected against tetanus, diphtheria and poliomyelitis.

In an attempt to clarify the situation regarding the available vaccines I have in the following section detailed the advantages and disadvantages of the commoner vaccines. I have listed the contra-indications to vaccination in an attempt to help readers decide when vaccination may or may not be suitable.

Since vaccinations cannot be performed without a doctor's authorisation it is important to discuss the suitability of a specific vaccine with the doctor concerned. You should make available any relevant medical information if the doctor is not your usual general practitioner. If you are not sure whether or not specific information is relevant then you should mention it anyway.

Vaccines: a quick guide

All vaccinations except for polio are generally given by injection; polio is usually given orally.

Vaccinations can be combined, and there are several double

and triple vaccines. Diphtheria can be combined with tetanus for example. Diphtheria, tetanus and pertussis may be given as a triple vaccine. (In some areas vaccination schedules may differ from those given below.)

Routine vaccinations

These following vaccines are normally given to provide general protection.

Diphtheria Children should be vaccinated against diphtheria at the age of three months and then again at six and twelve months. The vaccination is usually combined with the tetanus vaccination. Children over the age of 10 years who have not been vaccinated need to be tested for immunity before vaccination. There are no known circumstances where the diphtheria vaccination must be avoided.

Measles The measles vaccination is given to children in their second or third year. Vaccination is avoided if there is any history of fits, epilepsy or convulsions associated either with the child concerned or with his or her family. It should be avoided if there are any signs of physical underdevelopment, and if there is an allergy to the antibiotics neomycin or polymyxin (rarely prescribed) or to eggs (patients allergic to eggs develop general 'allergy' symptoms such as rashes, wheezes or vomiting.) If these contra-indications are ignored, reactions of various kinds can occur, convulsions being potentially the most serious.

Poliomyelitis All children should be vaccinated against polio at the age of three months and again at the ages of six and twelve months. An oral vaccine is usually given at the same time as the diphtheria and tetanus injection. Children should then be revaccinated at the age of 6 years, and on leaving school. Frequent travellers abroad should have booster doses every three years. Polio vaccination is avoided if there is diarrhoea and/or vomiting (to ensure full protection the symptoms must have subsided) or if there is any allergy to the antibiotics neomycin or polymyxin (rarely prescribed) or streptomycin.

Rubella (German measles) Girls should be vaccinated at the age off 11 whether or not they are thought to have had the disease, as diagnosis is often difficult. At least one month should elapse between rubella and TB injections. Patients allergic to rabbits, neomycin and polymyxin should avoid the vaccination.

Tetanus All children should be vaccinated at the age of three months and then again at six and twelve months, usually the vaccine is given along with the diphtheria and polio vaccines. A booster should be given when the child reaches the age of 6 and another when he or she leaves school. Children liable to sustain dirty wounds should have boosters every three years, otherwise boosters are only necessary on injury. You should not have more than one booster in any one year. If the vaccine is given too frequently there can be a reaction with a painful red swelling appearing at the injection site.

Tuberculosis At the age of 11 all children should be tested for TB immunity and if the reaction is negative they should be vaccinated (the vaccine is known as BCG). The disease is still prevalent in immigrant areas. Vaccination is avoided in cases of eczema or of local skin infections. The rubella (German measles) vaccination should be avoided for one month, and all other injections in the same arm for three months after the TB vaccination.

Whooping cough (pertussis) Whooping cough vaccination is usually given at three, six and twelve months along with diphtheria and tetanus. Whooping cough is the least effective of these three and some experts believe that there are serious risks involved in giving the vaccination. If there are any doubts the vaccination may be omitted. The vaccination is avoided if there is any history of fits, epilepsy or convulsions associated either with the child concerned or with his or her family. Similarly if there is any history of allergy (eczema, asthma, hay fever) or if your child has a fever, vaccinations should be avoided. There is a risk of brain damage if these contra-indications are ignored. If there is any severe local or general reaction to the first injection, further injections are probably best avoided.

Others

Cholera If you are travelling to Africa, the Middle East or the Far East, and occasionally if you are travelling to a Mediterranean country (check with your travel agent), you should be vaccinated against cholera. It is inadvisable for your children to have a cholera vaccination.

Infective hepatitis If you intend to live rough in a Third World country it may be worth asking your doctor to consider giving you a protective injection of immuno-globulin.

Influenza This vaccination is usually only given to adults at risk (such as sufferers of chronic bronchitis who would be in danger if they contracted flu). Influenza vaccination is avoided if the individual is allergic to eggs (see measles), and should only be given to children under the age of 9 years if they are suffering from a chronic lung or heart disease. In such cases a reduced dose of the vaccine is essential.

Smallpox Vaccination against smallpox is now unnecessary as the disease is officially extinct. If you are going abroad some countries will still ask for a certificate of vaccination but should be satisfied with a letter from your doctor.

Typhoid Travellers to most countries outside northern Europe and North America should be vaccinated; regular travellers should have a vaccination every three years. It is inadvisable for young children to have a typhoid vaccination.

Yellow fever Travellers to central Africa and South America should be vaccinated against yellow fever. Infants under the age of nine months should not have the vaccination, and it should not be given to people allergic to eggs (see measles) or to neomycin and polymyxin.

Appendix A:
Average height and weight tables for children

Mothers often worry about whether or not their children are tall enough, fat enough, thin enough or too tall. Subjective assessments whether made by well-meaning relatives, doctors or friends are of little value since the range of normal values is wide and the rate at which hormonal influences produce growth spurts is variable.

The two tables which follow are intended to provide readers with a rough and ready guide to the range within which normal, healthy children may fall. Average heights and weights (for what they are worth) can be estimated by simply finding the figure in the middle of the two extremes I have quoted.

Average height and weight

Girls

Age	Weight (lbs)	Length/Height (ins)
3 mon.	9-15	21-24
6 mon.	13-21	24-27
1 year	17-26	27-31
2 years	21-33	31-36
3 years	26-41	34-39
4 years	29-45	36-41
5 years	32-50	39-46
6 years	35-56	41-49
7 years	40-62	43-51
8 years	43-69	45-54
9 years	47-77	47-56
10 years	51-85	49-59
11 years	55-105	51-61
12 years	61-115	52-63
14 years	80-135	57-67
16 years	95-155	59-68

Boys

Age	Weight (lbs)	Length/height (ins)
3 mon.	9-15	22-25
6 mon.	14-22	24-28
1 year	19-28	28-32
2 years	22-34	32-37
3 years	26-39	34-41
4 years	29-44	37-43
5 years	32-50	40-46
6 years	36-55	41-48
7 years	39-63	43-51
8 years	42-70	45-53
9 years	46-80	47-56
10 years	50-89	48-58
11 years	55-97	51-60
12 years	63-108	52-63
14 years	75-135	56-68
16 years	95-155	61-73

Menstruation normally begins between the ages of 10 and 16.

Appendix B:
Is he developing fast enough?

All children develop at different rates and there is no such thing as a 'normal' rate of development. However, you should seek medical advice if:

By the time he reaches six months of age your child can't hold his head still and doesn't reach out for things with his hands.

By the time he reaches eighteen months of age he isn't walking by himself and making plenty of noises which may or may not be understandable.

By the time he reaches 2 years of age he can't produce any intelligible words and isn't playing with interest and enthusiasm.

If you are worried that he is not gaining height and weight at an appropriate rate.

If there is any problem then it is important that you ask for help as soon as possible. Even if your child's height and weight fall between the two extremes in the table in Appendix A you should seek advice if you are at all concerned.

Appendix C:
Tooth development

The first teeth usually appear at the age of about six months. The incisors at the front of the mouth invariably appear first, with the incisors in the lower jaw usually appearing before the incisors in the upper jaw.

By the age of 1 year there are usually teeth on each side of the incisors, in both the lower and upper jaws. The first molars, the large teeth at the back of the jaws, appear in the first few months of the child's second year of life. The canines, or eye teeth, fill in the gap between the incisors and the first molars by the time the child is about eighteen months of age. The second molars come at about or just after the age of 2 years.

Those first or milk teeth will usually last until your child reaches 6 or 8 years of age. Then the permanent teeth will start to appear. The first permanent teeth will probably be the incisors at the front of the mouth but the first set of permanent molars may appear at or around the same time. More incisors follow at about 8 or 9 years of age. By the time a child is 12 the premolars will have appeared between the molars, at the back of the mouth and the incisors at the front of the mouth. The canines come at about 12 to 14 years of age.

By the time they reach the age of 16 most children have their second molars right at the back of their mouths.

Finally the wisdom teeth, further back even than the second molars, appear at anything up to the mid-twenties.

Appendix D:
Weight conversion table

Pounds	Kilograms
1	0.45
2	0.9
5	2.25
10	4.5
50	22.5
100	45.0
150	67.5

Kilograms	Pounds
1	2.2
2	4.4
5	11.0
10	22.0
50	110.0

Appendix E:
Length-height conversion table

Inches	Centimetres
1	2.5
2	5.0
4	10.0
10	25.0
40	100.0
50	125.0

Centimetres	Inches
1	0.4
2	0.8
5	2.0
10	4.0
50	20.0
100	40.0

Appendix F:
Temperature conversion table

To convert Fahrenheit to centigrade subtract 32 from degrees F, multiply by 5 and divide by 9.

To convert centigrade to Fahrenheit multiply degrees centigrade by 9, divide by 5 and add 32.

Degrees Fahrenheit	Degrees centigrade	Degrees centigrade	Degrees Fahrenheit
95	35	35.0	95
96	35.6	35.5	95.9
97	36.1	36	96.8
98	36.7	36.5	97.7
99	37.2	37	98.6
100	37.8	37.5	99.5
101	38.3	38	100.4
102	38.9	38.5	101.3
103	39.4	39	102.2
104	40.0	39.5	103.1
105	40.6	40	104
106	41.1	40.5	104.9

Appendix G: Contact groups

Whether your child suffers from albinism or tuberous sclerosis, epilepsy or psoriasis, there will almost certainly be a society where you can meet parents with similar problems and share ideas and information. There are hundreds of small voluntary organisations in existence and you can find the address of your nearest group either by contacting your general practitioner or by asking at your local library.

Appendix H:
Keep a record!

When your children have measles or chickenpox you'll be convinced that you'll never forget the episode. When they have their first vaccinations you'll be certain you'll remember those too. But as the years go by those memories will fade. And you'll be uncertain about just what your child has had – and has not had. So, keep a simple record!

You can either fill in this chart here or copy it out into a notebook.

Child's name_____

Diseases contracted

	at age_____
_____	at age_____
_____	at age_____
_____	at age_____
_____	at age_____
_____	at age_____

Vaccinations

	date_____ date_____ date_____
_____	date_____ date_____ date_____
_____	date_____ date_____ date_____
_____	date_____ date_____ date_____
_____	date_____ date_____ date_____
_____	date_____ date_____ date_____

Allergies

	date_____
_____	date_____

Index